D1572836

IMMUNOLOGY AND AGEING

DEVELOPMENTS IN HEMATOLOGY AND IMMUNOLOGY

VOLUME 3

Also in this series:

1. Lijnen HR, Collen D and Verstraete M: Synthetic Substrates in Clinical Blood Coagulation Assays. 1980. ISBN 90-247-2409-0

2. Smit Sibinga C Th, Das PC and Forfar JO: Paediatrics and Blood Transfusion. 1982. ISBN 90-247-2619-0

Series ISBN 90-247-2432-5

IMMUNOLOGY AND AGEING

Proceedings of the Workshop held in Portonovo, Ancona, Italy,
September 25-26, 1980 as part of the EEC Concerted Action Programme on
Cellular Ageing and Decreased Functional Capacities of Organs

Sponsored by the Commission of the European Communities, as advised by the
Committee on Medical and Public Health Research

edited by

N. FABRIS
I.N.R.C.A. Gerontology Research Department,
Via Birarelli 8,
60100 Ancona,
Italy

1982

MARTINUS NIJHOFF PUBLISHERS
THE HAGUE / BOSTON / LONDON

FOR THE COMMISSION OF THE EUROPEAN COMMUNITIES

Distributors

for the United States and Canada
Kluwer Boston, Inc.
190 Old Derby Street
Hingham, MA 02043
USA

for all other countries
Kluwer Academic Publishers Group
Distribution Center
P.O. Box 322
3300 AH Dordrecht
The Netherlands

Library of Congress Cataloging in Publication Data

Main entry under title:

Immunology and ageing.

    (Developments in hematology and immunology ;
v. 3)
    1. Immunity--Congresses. 2. Aging--Immunological
aspects--Congresses. 3. Lymphatics--Aging--Con-
gresses. I. Fabris, N. II. EURAGE International
Workshop "Immunology and Aging" (1980 : Ancona,
Italy) III. Commission of the European Communities.
Committee on Medical and Public Health Research.
[DNLM: 1. Aging--Congresses. 2. Immunity--In old
age--Congresses. DE997VZK v.1 / WT 104 I336 1980]
QR185.3.I45   612'.67   82-2246

ISBN 90-247-2640-9   AACR2

ISBN 90-247-2640-9 (this volume)
ISBN 90-247-2432-5 (series)

Publication arranged by
Commission of the European Communities,
Directorate-General Information Market and Innovation,
Luxembourg

EUR 7619

PREFACE

The health status of the elderly and problems related to it are of
major importance for the European Community since at least 11% of the population is over 65 years of age. Social and medical advances will continue to promote the greying of the population in the member countries.
Increasing numbers of old people will reach older ages and this will, in
turn, call for increasing medical care and for a better understanding of
the biological aging processes which contribute to the development of many
diseases in the elderly population.

The increases in the number of older Europeans, in the incidence of diseases in this population and in the large monetary sums allocated to
health care of elderly persons have led to the establishment of a European programme in the discipline of biomedical gerontology. This programme, designated as EURAGE, is carried out as a "concerted action": its aim
is to promote the supranational coordination of research programmes performed within the member countries. An important aspect of the scientific
programme of EURAGE deals with the decline of immunity with age, which
is closely related to a number of clinical problems.

One of the means by which the coordination of European research in the
field of gerontology has been promoted is by the organisation of workshops.
This book records the papers presented at the EURAGE International workshop "Immunology and Ageing" which took place on September 25-26, 1980
in Portonovo, Ancona, Italy.

The success of the workshop was the result of the high caliber of the
presentations, the open and stimulating discussions and the organizational
abilities of Professor N. Fabris.

The papers presented by the members of Immunology group of EURAGE as well
as by experts from outside the EC provide a comprehensive evaluation of
the rapid developments in the field which may open new possibilities for
treatment and prevention of age-related immunological disorders.

D.L. Knook
Project Leader of EURAGE

CONTENTS

Preface

D.L. Knook   V

SESSION I: T- AND B-CELL ONTOGENY

A model for T-cell differentiation

O. Stutman   3

Alloantigens in human thymus

G.B. Ferrara, A. Longo, S. Eufrate, P. Musiani, L. Lauriola, M. Piantelli 17

Human thymocyte subsets: interleukins activity on mitogen responsiveness

H. Piantelli, L.Lauriola, G.G. Ferrara, P. Musiani   25

B- lymphocytes differentiation in adult human bone-marrow

G.C. De Gast   32

SESSION II: THE THYMIC MICROENVIRONMENT

Humoral function of the human thymus

R. Oosterom, L. Kater   37

Ultrastructual investigation of the lympho-epithelial and the lympho-me-
senchymal interactions in the ontogeny of the human thymus

B. von Gaudecker, H.K. Müller-Hermelink   51

Suppression of the antibody response induced by modified self is prevented by adult thymectomy. Restorative effect of facteur thymique serique

B. Grouix, D. Erard, J. Charreire, P. Galanaud   59

Effect of adenosine on non-histone chromatin proteins of thymocytes

A. Facchini, C.J.M. Leupers, L. Cocco, G.C.B. Astaldi, A.R. Mariani,
F.A. Manzoli, A. Astaldi   63

VIII

SESSION III: LYMPHOCYTE DISFUNCTIONS IN AGEING: EXPERIMENTAL APPROACH

Experimental immunogerontology: a perspective

D. Segre   71

T-helper, T-suppressor and B-cell functions in aging mice

M. Segre, J.J. Liu, D. Segre   78

Mouse T and B lymphocyte subpopulations: changes with age

J.J. Haaijman, J.M. Micklem   86

Effect of ageing and adult thymectomy (A-Tx) on primary syngeneic sensitization on monolayers of thyroid epitahelial cells (TEC)

J. Charreire   100

Increased occurrence of self reactive T cell clones in the aging immune
system

H. Schneider, H. Wekerle   110

Age-related changes in nude spleen cell function

R. Bösing-Schneider   116

Occurence of non viable lymphocytes and in vitro cytotoxic lymphocytes
in dying mice

P. Ebbesen, T. Faber, K. Fuursted   122

Analysis of lymphoid cell differentiation antigens in young and old chickens

G. Wick, K. Traill   125

Age dependence of T lymphocytes in altamurana's sheep

R. Celi, E. Jirillo, A. De Santis, G. Martemucci, P. Montemurro   130

SESSION IV: THYMIC ENDOCRINE ACTIVITY AND AGEING

Thymic hormones and aging

M. Dardenne, M.A. Bach, J.F. Bach   139

Enhanced helper activity in aging mice injected with thymic factors

D. Frasca, G. Doria   150

Thyroid-dependence of age-related decline of FTS production

N. Fabris, E. Mocchegiani, M. Muzzioli   156

SESSION V: IMMUNE DISFUNCTIONS IN AGED HUMANS

Immune senescence in man

M.L. Weksler   165

Autorosettes and autologous mixed lymphocytes reaction in human: two age-
  and sex-related models

C. Fournier, H.P. Chen, J. Charreire   187

Selective deficiency of T-lymphocytes subset(s) in aged and in Down's
syndrome subjects

C. Franceschi, F. Licastro, M. Chiricolo, M. Zannotti, N. Fabris,

E. Mocchegiani, L. Tabacchi, F. Barboni, M. Masi   195

Benign and malignant monoclonal gammopathy: differentiation by means of
the J chain

E.J.E.G. Bast, B. van Camp, R.E. Ballieux   200

CSF oligoclonal pattern in two cases of cerebral amyloid angiopathy

E. Schuller, R. Escouolle, F. Gray, H. Sager, J.J. Hauw   204

Polymorphonuclear functions in aging adult humans

J. Corberand, F. Nguyen, P. Laharrague, A.M. Fontanilles, B. Gleyzes,

E. Girard, C. Sénégas   211

Influence of supplemental oral zinc on the immune response of old people

J. Duchateau, G. Delespesse, M. Kunstler   220

SESSION I

T- AND B-CELL ONTOGENY

A MODEL FOR T CELL DIFFERENTIATION

O. Stutman

Cellular Immunology Section

Memorial Sloan-Kettering Cancer Center

New York, New York 10021, U.S.A.

ABSTRACT

A model for T cell development and renewal in the mouse that tries to incorporate commitment for T lineage (differentiation), development of repertoire for T cell interaction, regulation and function and T cell subset diversification is presented. The model includes prethymic, intrathymic and postthymic steps, regulated by thymic humoral factors, interaction between precursor and "inducer" cells and thymus-dependent products such as Interleukin-2. While commitment for T differentiation appear as pre and intrathymic events, both repertoire and subset specialization appear as intrathymic and postthymic events, the latter being preponderant. The relevance of developing a model for T cell development that may account for the complexities of modern day T cell sociology, in relation to the studies on the effects of aging on immune functions, is apparent.

INTRODUCTION

Two experimental facts are accepted concerning T cell development:
1) T cells are derived from hemopoietic stem cells which are influenced or "processed" by the thymus and 2) the thymus appears as an absolute requirement for differentiation of functional T cells (Stutman, 1975, 1977, 1978; Cantor & Weissman, 1976). The last statement implies that even in the seemingly thymus independent models to be discussed in the text, a thymus dependent product such as Interleukin-2 (IL-2) is required.

In the past five years a substantial amount of information and theory on the complexities of function, interaction and regulation of peripheral T cells has been incorporated into our immunological knowledge. The phenomenon of major histocompatibility (MHC) restriction of T cell function (Zinkernagel & Doherty, 1977; Zinkernagel, 1978; Katz, 1980), the ability to clearly define subsets of T cells with different functional properties (Cantor & Boyse, 1977) as well as the complex network regulations of immune reactivity (Jerne, 1975; Rajewsky & Eichmann, 1977; Binz & Wigzell, 1977; Cantor & Gershon, 1979), posed problems to the accepted models of T cell development. This conceptual problem, represented by the lack of a workable model for T cell renewal, also applied to the studies on the effects of aging on T cell functions, since most of the theoretical frameworks for such studies are based on models for T cell development which are either incomplete or too limited.

The importance of having a workable model for T cell development during ontogeny is that it may clarify the mechanism of daily cell renewal and maintenance of homeostatic levels of T cells in the periphery, and should include appropriate steps to account for irreversible commitment for the T lineage, development of repertoire of recognition units for physiological interactions and functional subspecialization into different T cell sets. It should be noted that based on life-span, estimates by isotopic labeling, as well as direct estimates of the cellular output in thymic veins of larger animals, approximately 5×10^5 cells/mg thymus/day are released into the blood via thymic veins (Joel et al., 1974). Using these values and the intrathymic data available, a figure for "daily replacement" can be obtained, which indicates the number of times per day that the thymic migrants can replace the circulating blood lymphocyte pool. It is interesting to note that despite the different techniques used, a value of approximately 3-5 was obtained in mice, guinea pigs and calves (see Joel et al,, 1974, for review). These impressive figures strongly indicate that no matter how sophisticated our knowledge of how one lymphocyte "speaks" to another or what a lymphocyte "sees" as antigen, it is important to develop a workable model for T cell development and replacement.

The demonstration of a population of immunologically competent T cells within the thymus (Blomgren & Andersson, 1969; Raff, 1971) was rapidly developed into a model of T cell differentiation based on the following sequence of events: stem cell → thymocyte → "mature" thymus lymphocyte → peripheral T lymphocyte (Raff, 1971, 1973). Thus, the whole process of differentiation was made intrathymic, and the "mature" thymus steroid-resistant lymphocyte was equated with the population of cells ready for export (Raff, 1971, 1973). This has been, and still is (as evidenced in Ledbetter et al., 1980, just to cite one recent example) the prevalent view of T cell development. However, such single lineage model has difficulty in explaining how diversification of functional subclasses of T cells appear or how the T cell repertoire is defined and refined. In addition, there are some actual experimental facts, such as the demonstration that the "mature" population of thymic lymphocytes is a resident population which is not exported (Stutman, 1977, 1978) and that the thymus exports steroid-sensitive postthymic precursors to the periphery (Stutman, 1975), which make the above mentioned model untenable.

An alternative hypothesis has been available since 1970, based on our own studies, which proposed that what the thymus actually exports after processing is not necessarily an immunologically competent T cell, but rather a "recognizable" committed precursor without detectable immune functions, termed "postthymic" (Stutman et al., 1969a, 1970 a,b; Stutman, 1975). This postthymic precursor (PTP) cell is an immunologically incompetent cell that displays surface antigens of the T lineage, and has a series of physical and functional characteristics which permitted its definition (Stutman, 1975, 1977, 1978; Stutman and Shen, 1979). Some of the distinct properties of PTP cells (as opposed to mature T cells) include: adherence to nylon wool, sensitivity to corticosteroids and expression of Thy 1 and Lyt 1, 2 & 3 surface antigens (Stutman, 1975, 1977, 1978; Stutman & Shen, 1979). Thus, further maturation in the periphery of the thymus-processed PTP cells, probably under the influence of thymic humoral factors, appears as one major pathway for the generation of competent T cells (Stutman, 1978; Stutman and Shen, 1979). Whether this circuit is the only one for replenishing the T cell pool, requires further study.

Thus, we proposed a model in which two major components could be defined: a) an intrathymic step for irreversible commitment of precursors of hemopoietic origin to the T lineage and b) an extrathymic step for further maturation and expansion of the PTP cells into immunologically competent T cells (Stutman, 1977, 1978). These two steps were also considered as part of the import-export function of the thymus usually termed "thymic traffic" (Stutman, 1977, 1978). In this model, the hemopoietic cells capable of migration to the thymus were operationally termed "prethymic" (Stutman et al., 1969a, 1970a,b; Stutman, 1975), and clearly include the "prothymocytes" defined by the in vitro induction studies and the repopulation of irradiated thymuses in vivo (Komuro et al., 1975; Scheid et al., 1978).

A brief comment on terminology. In our past publications we divided the process of T cell development into three steps: prethymic, intrathymic and postthymic (Stutman, 1977, 1978, 1979a,b). These three events are all related to the actual thymic processing of migrant cells of hemopoietic origin, via "thymus traffic" (Stutman, 1977, 1978). Thus, "postthymic" means thymus processed through an intrathymic step and subsequent export (Stutman, 1978). We reserve the term "extrathymic" for all the events

6

that, although possibly thymus dependent (via thymic humoral factors or
T cell-dependent products such as IL-2), do not include intrathymic processing. In some of our earlier publications, we also used prethymic and
postthymic in a different sense (Stutman et al., 1969a, 1970a,b). In general terms, and especially within the context of ontogeny, "prethymic"
meant any type of cell present before the appearance of the thymus in the
embryo. Thus, the only true prethymic hemopoietic cells would be the
early yolk sac cells, before the development of the thymus anlage, and
even these may be questioned, since such cells may be influenced by mater-
nal thymic humoral factors or thymus-dependent products such as IL-2.
Similarly, "postthymic" meant after the appearance of the thymus, including any type of thymic influence (Stutman et al., 1969a, 1970 a,b). We
feel that this latter terminology may create confusion (Stutman, 1978),
and we will use throughout the paper the terms as meant in the beginning
of this paragraph. However, semantics aside, the latter concept still
has some validity, since it is highly probable that all the hemopoietic
cells, whether or not enriched for "prothymocytes" (Scheid et al., 1978;
Komuro et al., 1975), used in most in vivo and in vitro studies may have
already received some form of thymic influence. This early thymic "priming or "imprinting" may also explain some of the results which suggest
T cell differentiation in absence of the thymus.

A MODEL FOR FUNCTIONAL T CELL DEVELOPMENT

In a previous publication we discussed a model for prethymic, intrathymic and postthymic events in T cell maturation (Stutman, 1978). These
processes combine differentiation, repertoire development and subspecialization, into a single intra- and postthymic chain of events (Stutman,
1978, 1979a,b). The present discussion will include a modified version,
incorporating the IL-2 circuit into the model. We use a general postulate that T cells are derived, under normal physiological conditions and
especially during early ontogeny, from hemopoietic precursor cells which
have migrated through the thymus, and that T cell functional development
requires thymus traffic as well as postthymic events, some of which may
also depend on thymic humoral factors.

"Circuit" is used to describe a possible self-regulatory system with
feedback for IL-2 production, as proposed for other regulatory systems
(Cantor and Gershon, 1979).

This new or modified model can be presented as a series of 12 points.

(1) Thymus processing, or products of thymus processed cells, are

obligatory for the generation of competent T cells.

(2) The prethymic step, represented by the development of the prothy-
mocyte compartment, is probably also thymus dependent, and influenced by
thymic humoral factors. Thus, there may be a thymus dependent "priming"
for lineage-commitment at the early prethymic precursor stage.

(3) Mature functional T cells in the periphery are mostly derived
from incompetent postthymic precursor (PTP) cells, most of which (if not
all) belong to the Lyt 123 class (Stutman, 1978). However, export of
other T cell types (Lyt 1), perhaps already functional, cannot be excluded
(Scollay & Weissman, 1980).

(4) Hemopoietic immigrants have 4 choices in the thymus:

a) become part of the exported precursor pool of PTP cells (which
also appears to be an heterogeneous compartment);

b) become part of the pool of thymocytes that die in situ (McPhee
et al., 1979) as part of the selective process described in points 8 to 10;

c) become part of the pool of intrathymic resident mature T cells
which are not exported (Stutman, 1978), this statement applies exclusively
to the steroid resistant population, and cannot include at present, other
mature intrathymic cells defined by other criteria (Mathieson et al., 1979;
London and Horton, 1980);

d) become Lyt 1 thymocytes (Mathieson et al., 1979) which may be
exported, and may give rise to the Lyt 1/IL-2 producing circuit in the
periphery (Stutman et al., 1980). It is also possible that Lyt 1 PTP-like
cells may be the precursors of the peripheral Lyt 1 cells involved in the
production of IL-2, either as producers or as inducers of production of IL-2
by other cells (Wagner & Rollinghoff,1978; Shaw et.al.,1980). The "antigen independent" production of IL-2 (i.e. independent of exogenous antigens) may be triggered via an "autologous mixed lymphocyte-like" response, in which Lyt 1 T cells
proliferate in response to Ia determinants on autologous macrophage-like cells.
(Lattime et al., 1980a,b).

(5) Contact of PRECURSOR with INDUCER cells which display appropriate
complementary surface determinants is necessary for functional T cell differentiation (Stutman, 1978).

(6) The inducer cells may impart 3 types of signals:a)irreversible commitment for T lineage;b)selection of appropriate dictionary of cell-interac-
tion units as part of the T cell repertoire and c)subspecialization into T subclasses. The first signal may be extrathymic,the second intrathymic,the
third signal postthymic (Stutman,1978).

(7) Without contact with inducer cells in the intrathymic environment, T cell precursors go into a pathway which generates non-functional T cells, or cells with abnormal (i.e. non-MHC restricted) function (Stutman, 1978).

(8) Excess thymocyte production within thymus is a selective process essential for functional development of T cells. The process of forming appropriate contacts between precursor and inducer cells may be probabilistic and the surplus cell production is necessary to achieve correct connections and compensate for development errors, as it happens in other biological systems (Stutman, 1978). Thus, theoretically one may propose that the precursor-inducer interactions include populations connected in a predictable manner, perhaps as complementary differentiation of "pairs" of cells (Stutman, 1978).

(9) These "matching" populations are regulated by genetic changes of 2 types: a) evolutionary changes in which the matching quality is not disrupted (concordant matching) and b) non-concordant changes which do not autonomously preserve the appropriate match (discordant matching).

(10) Thus, intrathymic selection would be for concordant matches (Stutman, 1978). The concordant matching would also generate cells capable of concordant interaction with appropriate matches in the periphery. The discordant matches will mean intrathymic death or, in some cases, malignant transformation (Stutman, 1978). This point implies that the precursor cells have to see within the thymic environment all the possible structures that they may find in periphery for the appropriate matches which lead to T cell subset development as well as associative recognition of MHC restricted nonself (Stutman, 1978; Zinkernagel, 1978; Katz, 1980). However, there is also evidence for additional refinement of recognition units in periphery, especially at the helper level (Zinkernagel, 1978; Lattime, et al., 1980c; Zinkernagel et al., 1980; Katz, 1980). It is possible that concordant selection is achieved via recognition of structures related to the MHC, or that the MHC is acting as a constant region for anchorage of other still undefined differentiation-directing molecules.

(11) The peripheral T cell pool in adult mice may be renewed by a combination of 3 types of events, though it is difficult as yet to quantitate their relative importance in producing each of the mature T cell types (Stutman, 1978). In addition, the magnitude of each component may be variable with age, i.e. in early ontogeny versus adult animals. The 3 probably non-exclusive mechanisms are:

a) continuing export from the thymus of either Lyt 123 PTP cells,

which are immature recognizable precursors, as well as Lyt 1 cells (probably more mature?);

b) expansion and differentiation of PTP cells in periphery, which
is dependent on thymic humoral factors of the "hormone" type;

c) peripheral expansion and differentiation of T cells, independent of thymic humoral factors, but dependent on other thymus-dependent
mediators of which IL-2 is the major example.

The last possibility, may appear at first glance to be "thymus independent." However, we emphasize that the recent examples of "thymus
independent" T cell differentiation (Kindred and Corley, 1977; Irle et al.,
1978; Gillis et al., 1979; Wagner et al., 1980; Galli and Droge, 1980),
though not involving the thymus per se or its secreted humoral factors,
have so far required either the use of products of mature thymus-processed
T cells or the presence of thymus processed or "thymus primed" precursor
cells. Thus, the putative "thymus independent" pathway is triggered by
"thymus dependent" products such as IL-2 or depends on the presence of
"thymus primed" cells.

(12) The experimental analysis of T cell development ought to distinguish carefully among 3 changes in the T cell populations, each of which
can affect the functional tests. These three changes are" a) "expansion"
of cell numbers without changes in cellular populations; b)"differentiation"
of one cell type into another with new and distinct properties (for example,
a cell might acquire the ability to receive the IL-2 signal and/or respond
to such signaling by dividing, etc.) and c) "activation" of a cell type,
which involves events which cause it to perform its function (for example,
binding to and killing a target cell, etc.). Thus, any specific mediator,
such as IL-2, whether produced by the thymus or not, could act on several
cell lineages or at several stages of a given lineage.

The strongest form of our model would be that the only role of the
intrathymic step is to generate the Lyt 1/IL-2 circuit in periphery, which
may be able to induce all of the mature T cell functions. In this absolute model, restriction would be learned in the periphery. On the other
hand, one of the "relative" forms of the model could propose that thymus
traffic and thymus dependent PTP expansion in periphery may build up the
precursor T cell pool, as well as the Lyt 1/IL-2 circuit, and that the
latter re ulates differentiation as well as activation of functional T
cells. Thus, functional activation of a T cell set may depend on "differentiation" via intrathymic and postthymic steps (as proposed in steps

4 and 6), as well as "activation" by the IL-2 second signal. There is no doubt that a large set of variations on this theme can also be proposed.

With the exception of the systems in which IL-2 is produced as a consequence of defined antigenic stimulation and acts as a "helper" or "T cell-replacing" factor (Watson et al., 1979), the physiological stimulus which triggers IL-2 production is still undefined (Moller, 1980). As we indicated in the beginning of the paper, we think that it is safe to postulate (2) possible triggering mechanisms: antigen independent and antigen dependent (this one may include the lectin-induction). These two mechanisms of IL-2 induction may be related to the differentiation versus the activation functions of IL-2, discussed in previous paragraphs. We will postulate that the physiological "antigen independent" triggering may be via an autologous mixed lymphocyte response, in which Lyt-1 cells respond with proliferation against Ia determinants on a syngeneic macrophage-like stimulator cell. We also have to add that "antigen independent" is understood as independent of an exogenous antigenic source.

In a previous study we demonstrated that the autologous or "syngeneic mixed lymphocyte reaction" (SMLR) was mediated by nylon wool non-adherent Lyt 1 spleen T cells which responded with proliferation to syngeneic nylon wool adherent cells (Lattime et al., 1980a). Further analysis demonstrated that the phenotype of the responder cell was Lyt 1^+, $2,3^-$, Qa 1^-, Ia$^-$ and that the stimulator cells belonged to a class of adherent, phagocytic Ia$^+$ cells (Lattime et al., 1980a,b).

We could also demonstrate that important amounts of IL-2 are produced as a consequence of the SMLR, and that the production of IL-2 is blocked by the same anti-Ia reagents that block SMLR (Lattime et al., 1980b; Stutman et al., 1980).

The SMLR responder cells belong to a category of long-lived T cells, since spleen cells derived from mice 8 months after adult thymectomy are still capable of responding in SMLR (Stutman et al., 1980). In addition, IL-2 is also produced during these responses (our unpublished results). These results support the view that once it is generated, the IL-2 circuit behaves as a relatively long-lived thymus-independent system.

In summary, it appears that IL-2 is produced in vitro (and possibly in vivo)by a mechanism which includes cells not immediately involved in a response to an exogenous antigen. It is obvious that questions such as the role of IL-2 in vivo; distant effects versus effects on neighbouring cells; differentiation versus activation of mature cells; regulation of

IL-2 production and action, etc. need extensive further studies. On the
other hand, the possibility that autoreactivity may serve as a critical
regulatory mechanism of the immune system is not new (Binz and Wigzell,
1978). In the present case we are proposing that an autoreactive reaction
may also be critical for the development and maintenance of the T cell
system.

On the other hand, the _in vivo_ role of the SMLR is still undefined.
Its possible _in vivo_ importance has been proposed via negative experiments,
i.e., the absence of SMLR responses in either NZB mice (Smith and Pasternak,
1978) or patients with lupus (Sakane et al., 1978), suggesting a link between autoimmune disease and capacity to produce SMLR, with SMLR as a loop
for the production of regulatory (suppressor) cells (Sakane et al., 1979).

If we accept the possible role of IL-2 in T cell development, we may
also have to postulate (2)possible ontogenic schemes: a) the first wave of
intrathymic T cells that matures in ontogeny is responsible for generating
an intrathymic SMLR-like response which produces IL-2 and begins the cycle
of T cell maturation (thus the only role of the thymic microenvironment is
to generate the first wave of T cells via humoral factors and cellular contacts and to present the appropriate Ia stimulus for the intrathymic SMLR)
and b) via thymus traffic and postthymic expansion a population of Lyt 1
responders to autologous Ia determinants is generated, which serves to
maintain the postthymic T cell pool in periphery. It is also apparent that
several other possibilities combining the above indicated extreme theories
can be proposed, with different degress of "thymus-dependent" and "IL-2-
dependent" stages. Thus, the intrathymic step may represent more of a
selective devise, rather than a site for actual lymphopoiesis.

The nature of the "inducer" cell, both in thymus and periphery required
for repertoire development and functional differentiation is not defined
(except for the suggestive evidence that in the thymus it may be in the
"radioresistant" portion of the thymic stroma, see Zinkernagel, 1978).
The characterization of the "inducer" cells and determination if they are
the same as the "restrictive" cell, appears to be important area for research. Perhaps the definition of the mechanics of the interactions between precursor and inducer cells may serve to clarify the mechanism of
restrictive recognition and the development of the T cell repertoire. In
addition and in relation to the age-dependent decline of T cell functions,
this model may explain the emergence of de-regulated autoimmune reactivity
with age. Thus, the inappropriate or defective function of the "inducer"

cells in the aging individual may generate cells that are either less functional or totally non-functional or, alternatively, that have abnormal reactivity. Thus, we may have to include the possible effects of senescence on the "inducer" cells both at intra and extrathymic locations, as important factors that determine the age-dependent decline of T cell functions or the abnormalities of regulatory T cell subsets. It is also apparent, from the previous discussion that the thymic humoral factors or thymic hormones appear to provide only a necessary but not sufficient signal for T cell differentiation and proliferation; a signal that in many cases is muddled by the biochemical heterogeneity of the thymic extracts (Stutman, 1980).

CONCLUSION

Although we all agree on the complexities of the T cell development, there is still a variety of opinions on the mechanisms of such process. This paper presents a re-statement of a theory aiming at explaining some of the particular features of T cell development and renewal. However, many questions are still _totally_ open concerning the proposed steps of T cell development.

Firstly, it is apparent that the thymic humoral factors, _per se_, are not the _only_ determinants of functional T cell development (Stutman, 1979a, 1980), and that T cell production and differentiation may be a consequence of a more complex pathway that includes, at least, the following stages: a) traffic of hemopoietic cells to the thymus; b) critical intrathymic steps that include humoral effects as well as cell-cell contacts between precursor and inducer cells, and also selective pressures for development of repertoire; c) export of selected postthymic precursors to the periphery; d) further maturation in the periphery, probably, but not exclusively, mediated by thymic humoral factors, but also requiring special cell-cell contacts for functional specialization; e) regulation of number and function via thymus-dependent soluble products such as IL-2 and f) complex interactions in the periphery between different subclasses of T cells and other cells, which regulate T cell function including "auto-reactive" responses.

Secondly, we also want to stress, again, that the magnitude of the different proposed steps of T cell development, under physiological conditions, cannot be ascertained at present writing. Similarly, we ignore the actual rate of age-dependent decay of the proposed steps.

Thirdly, the "absolute" form of our theory would make the thymus proper almost redundant once the IL-2 circuit has been generated. Such redundancy is not common in biological systems. Thus, we feel that the more integrated model, including any of the proposed "relative" forms of the theory may foster a better understanding of this complex system for cell renewal and differentiation.

Finally, why does an incomplete model persist? For quite a long time the clonal selection theory has dominated our immunological thinking. The theory was appealing mostly because it could account for a substantial amount of experimental results, otherwise unexplained. The theory gave somewhat of a "prokaryotic" view of the immune system, which was considered as a library of unrelated small immune systems or clones which were just waiting for antigen. After eliminating the forbidden clones during ontogeny, the surviving immunological receptors were thought to be directed mainly against non-self antigens. Furthermore, the whole process of selection for such clones was made intrathymic (see for example Jerne, 1971). Thus, the model of T cell development proposed at the beginning of this paper (i.e., Raff, 1971, 1973) seemed more than appropriate for such a system. Even the fact that there was experimental data contradicting the exclusive intrathymic instruction, such as the demonstration that depending on the strain combinations used, thymus grafts produced tolerance or not in thymectomized animals (Stutman et al., 1969b), did not affect the theory. The strict intrathymic selection approach would have predicted tolerance to the antigens presented within thymus in every instance (Jerne, 1971). However, a number of recent findings have changed the views of the immune system. Findings such as the positive and negative interactions between lymphoid cells, the role of idiotypes in the clonal interactions, the occurrence of compartments or subsets of T cells performing different functions and the MHC-restriction phenomenon strongly suggest the view that lymphocytes are not uncoupled wanderers, but have a mainly "eukaryotic" life: each lymphocyte speaks to some others and self-recognition is critically involved in the regulatory circuits of the immune system, via at least two types of receptors, one immunological for recognition of non-self and one physiological which recognizes membrane self-markers. What we are proposing here is a model for T cell renewal which addresses this complex cell to cell sociology. And, we are also requesting to those scientists involved in the age-dependent decline of the immune system, that they re-adjust their thinking towards these more comprehensive models of T and B cell renewal. There are probably many answers to the question at the beginning of this paragraph. The persistence of incomplete theories is probably the result of elaborate interactions between the initial value of the theory, its prestige, the wording used for the divulgation of the theory, the ease with which the theory explained the findings of the individual scientists and finally, a certain degree of intellectual laziness.

ACKNOWLEDGMENT

The experimental work described was supported by NIH grants CA-08748, CA-15988, CA-17818, CA-25932, AG-02479 and AG-02152. I thank Drs. E. Lattime, R. Miller and S. Macphail for discussion and sharing of results and Ms. L. Stevenson for preparation of this manuscript.

REFERENCES

Binz, H. and Wigzell, H.: Antigen-binding, idiotypic T-lymphocyte receptors. Contemp. Topics Immunobiol. 7: 113-177, 1977.
Binz, H. and Wigzell, H.: Horror Autotoxicus? Fed. Proc. 37: 2365-2369, 1978.
Blomgren, H. and Andersson, G.: Evidence for a small pool of immunocompetent cells in the mouse thymus. Exp. Cell Res. 57: 185-192, 1969.
Cantor, H. and Boyse, E.: Regulation of the immune response by T-cell subclasses. Contemp. Topics. Immunobiol. 7: 47-67, 1977.
Cantor, H. and Gershon, R.K.: Immunological circuits: cellular composition. Fed. Proc. 38: 2058-2064, 1979.
Cantor, H. and Weissman, I.: Development and functions of subpopulations of thymocytes and T lymphocytes. Progr. Allergy 20: 1-64, 1976.
Galli, P. and Droge, W.: Development of cytotoxic T lymphocyte precursors in the absence of the thymus. Eur. J. Immunol. 10: 87-92, 1980.
Gillis, S., Union, N.A., Baker, P.E. and Smith, K.A.: The in vitro generation and sustained culture of nude mouse cytolytic T-lymphocytes. J. Exp. Med. 149: 1460-1476, 1979.
Irle, C., Piguet, P.F., and Vassalli, P.: In vitro maturation of immature thymocytes into immunocompetent T cells in the absence of direct thymic influence. J. Exp. Med. 148: 32-45, 1978.
Jerne, N.K.: The somatic generation of immune recognition. Eur. J. Immunol. 1: 1-9, 1971.
Jerne, N.K.: The immune system: a web of V domains. Harvey Lect. 70: 93-110, 1975.
Joel, D.D., Chanana, A.D. and Cronkite, E.P.: Thymus cell migration. Ser. Haematol. 7: 464-481, 1974.
Katz, D.H.: Adaptive differentiation of lymphocytes: Theoretical implications for mechanisms of cell-cell recognition and regulation of immune responses. Adv. Immunol. 29: 137-207, 1980.
Kindred, G., and Corley, R.B.: A T cell-relacing factor specific for histocompatibility antigens in mice. Nature (Lond.) 268: 531-532, 1977.
Komuro, K., Goldstein, G. and Boyse, E.A.: Thymus-repopulating capacity of cells that can be induced to differentiate to T cells in vitro. J.

Immunol. 115: 195-198, 1975.

Lattime, E.C., Golub, S.H. and Stutman, O.: Lyt-1 cells respond to Ia-bearing macrophages in the murine syngeneic mixed lymphocyte reaction. Eur. J. Immunol. 10: 723-726, 1980a.

Lattime, E.C., Gillis, S., David, C., Stutman, O.: Interleukin-2, production in the syngeneic mixed lymphocyte reaction. Eur. J. Immunol., 1980b, in press.

Lattime, E.C., Gerhson, H.E. and Stutman, O.: Allogeneic radiation chimeras respond to TNP-modified donor and host targets. J. Immunol. 124: 274-278, 1980c.

Ledbetter, J.A., Rouse, R.V., Micklem, H.S. and Herzenberg, L.A.: T cell subsets defined by expression of Lyt 1,2,3 and Thy-1 antigens. Two-parameter immunofluorescence and cytotoxicity analysis with monoclonal antibodies modifies current views. J. Exp. Med. 152: 280-295,1980.

London, J. and Horton, M.A.: Peanut Agglutinin. V. Thymocyte subpopulation in the mouse studied with peanut agglutinin and Lyt-6.2 antiserum. J. Immunol. 124: 1803-1807, 1980.

Mathieson, B.J., Sharrow, S.O., Campbell, P.S. and Asofsky, R.: An Lyt differentiated thymocyte subpopulation detected by flow microfluorometry. Nature 277: 478-480, 1979.

McPhee, D., Pye, J. and Shortman, K.: The differentiation of T lymphocytes. V. Evidence for intrathymic death of most thymocytes. Thymus 1: 135-193, 1979.

Moller, G., Ed.: T cell stimulating growth factors. Immunol. Rev. 51: 1980.

Raff, M.C.: Evidence for a subpopulation of mature lymphocytes within mouse thymus. Nature New Biol. (London) 229: 182-183, 1971

Raff, M.C.: T and B lymphocytes and immune responses. Nature (London) 242: 19-23, 1973.

Rajewsky, K. and Eichmann, K.: Antigen receptors of helper T cells. Contemp. Topics Immunobiol. 7: 69-112, 1977.

Sakane, T., Steinberg, A.D. and Green, I.: Failure of autologous mixed lymphocyte reactions between T and non-T cells in patients with systemic lupus erythematosus. Proc. Natl. Acad. Sci. USA 75: 3464-3468, 1978.

Sakane, T. and Green, I.: Specificity and suppressor function of human T cells responsive to autologous non-T cells. J. Immunol. 123: 584-589, 1979.

Scheid, M.P., Goldstein, G., Boyse, E.A.: The generation and regulation of lymphocyte populations, Evidence from differentiative induction systems in vitro. J. Exp. Med. 147: 1727-1743, 1978.

Scollay R. and Weissman, I.L.: T cell maturation: Thymocyte and thymus migrant populations defined with monoclonal antibodies to the antigens Lyt-1, Lyt-2 and ThB. J. Immunol. 124: 2841-2844, 1980.

Shaw, J., Caplan, B., Paetkau, V., Pilarski, L.M., Delovitch, T. and McKenzie, I.F.C.: Cellular origins of co-stimulator (IL-2) and its activity in cytotoxic T lymphocyte responses. J. Immunol. 124: 2231-2239, 1980.

Smith, J.B. and Pasternak, R.D.: Syngeneic mixed lymphocyte reaction in mice: Strain distribution, kinetics, participating cells and absence in NZB mice. J. Immunol. 121: 1889-1892, 1978.

Stutman, O.: Humoral thymic factors influencing possthymic cells. Ann. N.Y. Acad. Sci. 249: 89-105, 1975.

Stutman, O.: Two main features of T cell development: thymus traffic and postthymic maturation. Contemp. Topics Immunobiol. 7: 1-46, 1977.

Stutman, O.: Intrathymic and extrathymic T cell maturation. Immunol. Rev. 42: 138-184, 1978.

16

Stutman, O.: Cellular and humoral requirements for T cell development. Ann. N.Y. Acad. Sci. 332: 123-127, 1979a.

Stutman, O.: Development of T cells in the mouse, in T and B lymphocytes: Recognition and Function. Ed. F.H. Bach, B. Bonavida, E.S. Vitetta and C.F. Fox, pp. 77-85 (Academic Press, N.Y., 1979b).

Stutman, O.: Thymic hormones and T cell development. Immunological Aspects of Aging. Ed. D. Segre and L. Smith, in press. (Marcel Dekker, Inc., N.Y., 1980).

Stutman, O. and Shen, F.W.: Postthymic precursor cells give rise to both Lyt-1 and Lyt-23 subsets of T cells. Transplant. Proc. 11: 907-909, 1979.

Stutman, O., Yunis, E.J. and Good, R.A.: Carcinogen-induced tumors of the thymus. IV. Humoral influences of normal thymus and functional thymomas and influence of post-thymectomy periods on restoration. J. Exp. Med. 130: 809-819, 1969a.

Stutman, O., Yunis, E.J. and Good, R.A.: Tolerance induction with thymus grafts in neonatally thymectomized mice. J. Immunol. 103: 92-99, 1969b.

Stutman, O., Yunis, E.J. and Good, R.A.: Studies on thymus function. I. Cooperative effect of thymic function and lymphohemopoietic cells in restoration of neonatally thymectomized mice. J. Exp. Med. 132: 583-600, 1970a.

Stutman, O., Yunis, E.J. and Good, R.A.: Studies on thymus function. II. Cooperative effect of newborn and embryonic hemopoietic liver cells with thymus function. J. Exp. Med. 132: 601-612, 1970b.

Stutman, O., Lattime, E.C., Gillis, S. and Miller, R.A.: Role of Interleukin-2 in postthymic maturation of T cells. Behring Inst. Mitt. 67: 95-104, 1980.

Wagner, H. and Rollinghoff, M.: T-T cell interactions during in vitro cytotoxic allograft responses. I. Soluble products from activated Ly 1 T cells trigger autonomously antigen-primed Ly 23 cells to proliferation and cytolytic activity. J. Exp. Med. 148: 1523-1538, 1978.

Wagner, H., Hardet, C., Heeg, K., Rollinghoff, M. and Pfizenmaier, K.: T cell derived helper factor allows in vivo induction of cytotoxic T cells in nu/nu mice. Nature (Lond.) 284: 278-279, 1980.

Watson, J.D., Gillis, S., Marbrook, J., Mochizuki, D. and Smith, K.A.: Biochemical and biological characterization of lymphocyte regulatory molecules. I. Purification of a class of murine lymphokines. J. Exp. Med. 150: 849-861, 1979.

Zinkernagel, R.M.: Thymus and lymphoreticular cells: their role in T cell maturaiton in selection of T cells H2-restrictions-specificity and H2 linked Ir gene control. Immunol. Rev. 42: 224-270, 1978.

Zinkernagel, R.M. and Doherty, P.C.: Major transplantation antigens, viruses and specificity of surveillance T cells. Contemp. Topics Immunobiol. 7: 179-220, 1977.

Zinkernagel, R.M., Althage, A., Waterfield, E., Kindred, B., Welsh, R.M., Callahan, G. and Pincetl, P.: Restriction specificities, alloreactivity and allotolerance expressed by T cells from nude mice reconstituted with H2-compatible or incompatible thymus grafts. J. Exp. Med. 151: 376-399, 1980.

ALLOANTIGENS IN HUMAN THYMUS

Giovanni B. Ferrara [+], Anna Longo [+], Sergio Eufrate [X], Pietro Musiani[o],

Libero Lauriola [o] and Mauro Piantelli [o].

[+]Immunohematology Research Center and [X] Pediatric Cardiosurgery

Department, Ospedale Gen. Prov. Massa, A.V.I.S., Bergamo,

and [o] Pathology Department, Università Cattolica

R O M A - Italy

ABSTRACT

26 alloantisera obtained by planned immunization involving HLA-A and HLA-B compatible individuals were tested for their complement-mediated cytotoxic activity against peripheral blood T cells (PBT) and thymocytes from 15 patients. Of the 7 active alloantisera only Fe 11/23 anti-serum recognized antigens mainly present on PBT whereas the remaining 6 antisera showed spedicicity against antigens preferentially expressed on thymocytes. In this last group there are 2 sera (Fe 137/15, Fe 81/11) preferentially reacting with the immature cortical PNA+ or with the mature medullary PNA-fraction respectively. The Fe 128/18 serum recognized antigens mainly expressed on T_M depleted preparations from both PNA+ and PNA- subsets. Only the Fe 137/15 reacted with the vast majority of PNA+ cells. The reactivity of the antisera against the majority but not all of the thymuses studied auggests that they recognized a polymorphic membrane component.

INTRODUCTION

Thymocyte subsets can be identified on the basis of their differing agglutinability by peanut agglutinin (PNA). PNA+ cells, mainly located in the cortex, are immature cells as judged by their responsiveness to mitogens and to alloantigens. Conversely the PNA- subset is composed of medullary, relatively mature cells (Reisner, et al., 1979). More recently we found that in both cortex and medulla there is a distinct subset with Fc-IgM receptors (T_M cells); moreover it was also found that only T_M medullary cells were able to respond to mitogens (Musiani, et al., 1980.

Recently antisera obtained from HLA-A and B compatible individuals who had undergone a planned immunization program were shown to contain specific anti-PBT activity (Ferrara, et al., 1979). The reactivity of these antisera against some but not all members of a given population indicates that they recognize a polymorphic cell surface component (Ferrara, et al., 1980).

Aim of this study was to investigate the alloantisera reactivity against PBT cells and thymocytes obtained from the same individuals. The presence of alloantigens preferentially expressed on cortical or medullary thymocyte subsets characterized by different maturative steps was detected.

MATERIALS AND METHODS

Volunteers for immunization were selected from blood donors (A.V.I.S., Bergamo, Italy) and typed for all known specificities of HLA-A,B, C and DR loci with sera obtained from VI and VII Histocompatibility Workshops. The standardized immunization procedure and the measures taken to avoid possible harmful effects have been described in detail elsewhere (Ferrara, et al., 1978).

PBT cells forming rosettes with neuraminidase-treated sheep erythrocytes were isolated from plastic nonadherent mononuclear cells by Ficoll-Hypaque density gradient centrifugation.

Thymocyte suspensions were obtained from 15 young patients undergoing open heart surgery.

In 7 cases PNA+ and PNA- subsets were obtained by differential agglutination by peanut agglutinin following the procedure reported by Reisner et al. (1979). PNA was purified from fresh peanuts using a sialic acidless fetuin-sepharose colum (Irlé, 1977).

Detailed description of the procedure employed for the separation of T_M thymocytes were recently reported by us (Carbone, et al., 1979) Musiani, et al., in press).

Microcytotoxicity test was performed according to the method described by Van Rood et al. (1976), omitting the staining by anti-human immunoglobulin. To check the dilution to be used for testing the antisera under study, rabbit complement was titred against each thymocyte preparation with 2 antisera: a polyspecific anti-HLA reacting against more than 95% of PBT and the Fe 137/15 serum. Anti-T cell alloantisera were previously tested for their C-mediated cytotoxic capacity against PBT from both specific donor and recipient. Titration curves showed that most of these anti sera, although highly specific for T cells (Ferrara, 1979), gave optimal reactions when used undiluted. No additional Killing could be detected when cells were reexposed to a given alloantiserum and complement.

RESULTS

Seven out 26 alloantisera exhibited cytotoxic activity against either thymocytes or PBT. Only Fe 11/23 serum was shown to recognized antigens mainly present on PBT (data not shown). On the other hand, the remai
ning 6 alloantisera showed specificity against antigens preferentially ex
pressed on thymocytes (Table 1). In this last group are 2 sera (Fe 137/15;
Fe 81/11) characterizd by preferential reactivity with PNA$^+$ or PNA$^-$ cells
respectively (Table 2). The Fe 129/18 alloantiserum, reacting with cells
present in both PNA$^+$ and PNA$^-$ fractions (see Table 2), recognized antigens preferentially expressed on T_M depleted subsets while the Fe 81/11
mainly reacted with T_M depleted subset of PNA$^-$ fraction (Table 3).

DISCUSSION

Data in this paper indicate that alloantisera from planned immunization may exhibit specific activity against thymocytes and PBT obtained
from the same subjects. Since variable percentages of reactivity were obtained by testing different antisera against a thymocyte preparation from
a single subject it is lukely that the antisera contain antibodies against various antigenic specificities or that cross-reacitivity exists in
tha antigenic system recognized. The reactivity of the antisera considered against the majority but not all of the thymuses could indicate that
they recognize a polymorphic surface membrane component.

Moreover thymocyte subsets at different maturative stages can be distinguished on the basis of their different reactivity with alloantisera.
For example, Fe 137/15 recognized antigens expressed on cortical immunocompetent PNA$^+$ cells while Fe 81/11 reacted preferentially with medullary,
immunoincompetent, PNA$^-$ thymocytes.

Of particular interest is the preferential reactivity of Fe 128/18 against
T_M depleted preparations from both thymic cortec and medulla given its
prebiously demonstrated preferential reactivity with peripheral T_G cells
, (Ferrara, et al., 1980). Thus it is possible that a common antigen is expressed by peripheral T_G cells and fraction of T_M depleted thymocytes;
Fc-IgG receptor could than be acquired at the lymphoid periphery by post-
-thymic precursor cells derived from non-T_M thymocytes.

Owing to the planned immunization program almost all antisera contain anti-DR specificities; nevertheless the presence of anti-DR antibodies
is absolutely indipendent of the observed anti-thymocyte activity since

Dr-determinants are absent on thymic lymphocytes (Janossy et al., 1980).

Fe 137/15, unreactive with PBT is cytotoxic for the majority of thy-mocytes and for almost all cortical cells. Recently McMichael et al., (1979) obtained a monoclonal antibody difining a surface antigen (HTA) ex-clusively expressed by the majority (85%) of HLA-negative thymocytes. The reciprocal expression of HTA1 with HLA is simalar to those of the mouse TL antigens (Konda et al., 1973). Owing to the lack of HLA-antigens on human cortical cells (Janossy et al., 1980), the reactivity of anti-HTA1 monoclo nal antibody with immature thymocytes is similar to that of Fe 137/15 allo antiserum.

Finally, how is it possible to obtain antibodies against antigens pre sent an thymocytes but absent on PBT by immunizing with PBT cells? One could suppose that the planned immunization procedure triggers an in vivo two way mixed lymphocyte reaction so that antibodies against activated lymphocytes can be stimulated. Supporting this view are very recent data showing that polymorphic, HLA linked determinants detectable on lecting activated T cells are not expressed by resting PBT. These determinants are encoded in the HLA-A region and may represent the human counterpart of the TL A region determinants of the mouse (Gazit et al., 1980).

This work was supported in part by Progetto Finalizzato C.N.R. "Controllo della Crescita Neoplastica".

TABLE 1

ALLOANTISERA RECOGNIZING ANTIGENS PREFERENTIALLY EXPRESSED ON THYMOCYTES

Alloantiserum	Fe 81/11		Fe 141/16		Fe 127/6		Fe 137/15		Fe 153/5		Fe 118/9	
Donor	PBT	Thymocytes	PBT	Thymocytes	PBT	Thymocytes	PBT	Thymocytes	PBT	Thymocytes	PBT	Thymocytes
C.B.	0	31	1	32	6	53	0	63	12	47	17	59
C.S.	3	47	0	5	6	51	0	61	1	5	3	51
S.M.	8	32	2	37	2	4	5	26	6	36	0	42
G.D.	5	49	4	16	2	64	2	70	8	0	2	63
P.S.	7	16	5	10	9	29	18	77	8	18	11	34
C.A.	11	37	9	12	0	28	9	86	1	8	1	60
C.C.	6	24	0	41	6	33	8	74	0	47	0	31
F.G.	2	20	9	35	11	30	14	66	10	30	1	31
V.S.	0	23	0	27	7	39	3	68	0	26	1	43
D.S.M.	0	16	3	17	4	23	2	100	8	18	6	14
C.G.	2	18	2	24	8	44	2	74	4	13	9	43
G.C.	5	15	0	6	11	15	1	73	0	22	6	33
U.S.	2	27	5	4	8	37	8	61	9	24	2	24
M.I.	0	10	4	12	6	29	5	71	2	24	9	25
R.M.	9	36	5	32	6	41	19	84	2	33	11	65

THE VALUES ARE EXPRESSED AS PERCENTAGES OF PERIPHERAL T LYMPHOCYTES OR THYMOCYTES.

TABLE 2

ALLOANTISERA RECOGNIZING ANTIGENS PREFERENTIALLY EXPRESSED ON SUBSETS DEFINED BY THE PEANUT LECTIN
AGGLUTINATING CAPACITY

Alloantiserum	PBT-cells	Thymocytes	PNA$^+$ a) thymocytes	PNA$^-$ b) thymocytes	Donor
Fe 81/11	0	31	7	28	C.B.
	7	19	0	24	S.V.
	6	24	5	22	C.C.
	11	37	4	7	C.A.
	9	24	3	26	S.F.
	2	20	6	18	F.G.
	0	10	2	17	M.I.
Fe 137/15	0	63	100	47	C.B.
	11	78	100	48	S.V.
	8	74	77	45	C.C.
	9	86	81	50	C.A.
	14	88	100	51	S.F.
	14	66	83	45	F.G.
	5	71	77	42	M.I.
Fe 129/18	23	40	47	28	C.B.
	19	27	0	39	S.V.
	16	51	39	34	C.C.
	6	49	22	23	C.A.
	7	19	26	24	S.F.
	2	31	29	20	F.G.
	9	20	21	32	M.I.

a) PNA$^+$ thymocytes: peanut lectin positive, immunoincompetent and "immature" cortical thymocytes.

b) PNA$^-$ thymocytes: peanut lectin negative, immunocompetent and "mature" medullary thymocytes.

THE VALUES ARE EXPRESSED AS PERCENTAGES OF PERIPHERAL T LYMPHOCYTES OR THYMOCYTES.

TABLE 3

ALLOANTISERA RECOGNIZING ANTIGENS PREFERENTIALLY EXPRESSED ON A SUBSET OF THYMOCYTES

Alloantiserum	PBT-cells	Thymocytes	PNA⁺	PNA⁺, T_M⁻ enriched	PNA⁺, T_M⁻ depleted	PNA⁻	PNA⁻, T_M⁻ enriched	PNA⁻, T_M⁻ depleted	Donor
Fe 61/1:	0	31	7	8	20	28	5	39	C.B.
	11	37	4	4	0	17	5	25	C.A.
	6	24	5	3	14	22	1	33	C.C.
Fe 129/18	23	40	47	16	39	18	18	43	C.B.
	6	49	22	3	14	23	12	32	C.A.
	16	51	39	1	35	34	7	43	C.C.

THE VALUES ARE EXPRESSED AS PERCENTAGES OF PERIPHERAL T LYMPHOCYTES OR THYMOCYTES.

24

References

Carbone, A., Piantelli, M., Musiani, P., Pozzuoli, R. and L. Lauriola. 1979. Fc receptor for IgM: Factors influencing detection on human T lymphocytes. J. Immunol.. Methods 29:245.

Ferrara, G.B., 1979. Identification of new cell surface markers in man: The problem of immunogenicity. Transplantation Proceedings XI:715.

Ferrara, G.B., Longo, A., Colombatti, M., and Moretta, L.. 1980. Alloantigens of human T-cell subsets. In Thymic hormones and T lymphocytes. Edited by F. Aiuti and H. Wigzell. Academic Press, London.

Ferrara, G.B., Strelkauskas, A.J., Longo, A., McDowel, J., Yunis, E.J., and Schlossman, J.F.. 1979. Markers of human T cell subsets identified by alloantisera. J. Immunol. 123:1272.

Ferrara, G.B., Tosi, R., Longo, A. Castellani, A., Viviani, C. and Carnati, G.. 1978. Safe blood transfusion procedure for immunization against MHC determinants in man. Transplantation 26:150.

Gazit, E., Terhorst, C., and Yunis, E.J., 1980. The human "T" genetic region of the HLA linkage group is a polymorphism detected on lectin-activated lymphocytes. Nature, 284:275.

Irlé, C., 1977. Rapid purification of peanut agglutinin by sialic acidless fetuin-sepharose column. J. Immunol.. Methods 17:1170.

Janossy, G., Thomas, J.A., Bollum, F.J., Granger, S., Pizzolo, G., Bradstock, K.F., Wong, L., McMichael, A., Geneshaguru, K., and Hoffbrand, A.V., 1980. The human thymic microenvironment: an immunohistologic study. J. Immunol. 125:202.

Konda, S., Stockert, E., and Smith, R.T., 1973. Immunologic properties of mouse thymus cells: membrane antigen patterns associated with various cell subpopulations. Cell. Immunol. 7:275.

McMichael; A.J., Pilch, J.R., Galfre, G., Mason, D.Y., Fabre, J.W., and Milstein, C., 1979. A human thymocyte antigen defined by a hybrid myeloma monoclonal antibody. Eur. J. Immunol. 9:205.

Musiani, P., Lauriola, L., Carbone, A., Maggiano, N., and Piantelli, M., Lymphocyte subsets in human thymus: expression of IgM-Fc receptor by peanut agglutinin positive and negative thymocytes. Thymus, in press.

Reisner, Y., Biniaminov, M., Rosenthal, E., Sharon, N., and Ramot, B., 1979. Interaction of peanut agglutinin with normal human lymphocytes and with leukemic cells. Proc. Natl. Acad. Sci. USA. 76:447.

Van Rood, J.J., Van Leeuwen, A., and Ploem, J.S., 1976. Simultaneous detection of two cell populations by two-colour fluorescence and application of the recognition of B-cell determinants. Nature 262:795.

HUMAN THYMOCYTE SUBSETS: INTERLEUKINS ACTIVITY ON MITOGEN RESPONSIVENESS

M. Piantelli, L. Lauriola, G.B. Ferrara and P. Musiani

Pathology Department, Università Cattolica, Roma; Centro Ricerche Immunoematologiche, Ospedale, Massa; A.V.I.S., Bergamo; ITALY.

ABSTRACT

Conditioned media from LPS stimulated human macrophages (IL1) and from PHA stimulated PNA$^-$ thymocytes (IL2) were obtained. The very poor proliferative responses to PHA exhibited by the PNA$^+$, cortical thymocytes can not be significantly enhanced either increasing cellular density or by adding IL1, IL2 or both. On the contrary PNA$^-$, medullary thymocytes respond vigorously; furthermore their response can be augmented either by increasing the cellular density or by adding IL1, IL2 or both. The responding subset within the PNA$^-$ thymocytes is mainly constituted by cells bearing Fc-IgM receptors. Our data indicate that: - PNA$^-$ thymocytes are able to produce IL2. - The most advanced intrathymic maturative step is attained by PNA$^-$ T_M medullary cells. - IL2 alone can increase the blastic proliferation of PNA$^-$ cells but the highest mitogenic responses are obtained by the synergistic action of IL1 and IL2.

INTRODUCTION

The proliferation of T lymphocytes in response to phytomitogens and antigens is often taken as a proof for immunocompetence. In human thymus are distinct subsets differing in their reactivity to mitogens. It has been demonstated that although the majority of cortical, peanut lectin agglutinable (PNA$^+$) thymus cells are relatively deficient in their response to various mitogenic stimuli, the minor medullary, peanut lectin unagglutinable (PNA$^-$)

subpopulation responds vigorously to phytomitogens and to allogeneic lymphocytes (Reisner, et al., 1979). Recently, we found that in both cortex and medulla of human thymus there is a distinct subset characterized by membrane surface receptors for the Fc portion of IgM (T_M cells) (Musiani, et al. 1980). Moreover it was also observed that only T_M medullary thymocytes were able to respond to PHA(Musiani et al., in press).

At the Second International Lymphokine Workshop a consensus was reached with regard to the definition of two factors which modulate lymphocyte activation (Mizel and Farrar, 1979). Both of these factors enhance the thymocyte blastic responses. Interleukin 1 (IL1), originally designated lymphocyte activating factor, is produced by macrophages while interleukin 2 (IL2, T cell growth factor) production requires T cells and macrophages.

This work deals with the analysis of the IL1 and IL2 activity on the blastic responses to PHA exhibited by different human thymocyte subsets.

MATERIALS AND METHODS

Thymocytes were separated in two subpopulation by agglutination with peanut agglutinin (PNA) according to the procedure reported by Reisner et al., (1979). PNA was purified following the method described by Irlè, (1977). In order to perform FITC-PNA binding assay, thymocytes (0.1 ml, $3 \cdot 10^6$ cells) were incubated with FITC-PNA (0.1 ml, 350µg/ml) for 20 min at room temperature. T_M thymocytes were identified by rosetting with IgM - coated ox erythrocytes and were separated from the non rosetting fraction on Ficoll-Hypaque density gradient (Musiani, et al., 1980).

Thymocyte cultures were established in microtitre flat-bottomed plates in triplicate and consisted of 0.2 ml of culture medium containing 1×10^5 or 5×10^6 cells. In some experiment cells were coltured in the presence of 15% IL1 and 35% IL2. PHA was added at 5 μg/ml. Cultures were incubated for 88 hr in a 5% humidified environment; 16 hr before the end of the incubation period, 0.5 μ Ci (Methyl-^{3}H) thymidine (5 Ci/mmole; Amersham, England) were added to each culture well. The cultures were then harvested for scintillation spectrometry.

IL1 was obtained from LPS stimulated human peripheral blood adherent cells (Blyden and Handschumacker, 1977). IL2 was prepared by stimulating PNA$^-$ thymocytes ($2\cdot10^6$/ml) with PHA (2.5 μg/ml) for 48hr.IL2 activity was determined according to the procedure reported by Gillis et al.,(1978).

RESULTS

In the ten thymocyte suspensions in which the separation by PNA was performed 79.1$\pm$3% (mean $\pm$ S.D.) of the cells were FITC-PNA$^+$ while approximately 65% of the thymocytes were agglutinated by the lectin. The agglutinated cells were virtually all (98%) FITC-PNA$^+$; howerer the non-agglutinated fraction contained about 1/3 of weakly FITC-PNA$^+$ cells. T_M cells accounted for 24$\pm$4% in PNA agglutinable fraction and for 33$\pm$3% in PNA non-agglutinable subset.

Results concerning the proliferative responses of the various thymocyte subsest are shown in Table 1.

TABLE I: Mitogenic response to PHA of thymocyte subsets*

Thymocyte fraction:	Cells: 0.5×10^6/ml	Cells: 2.5×10^6/ml
Unseparated	3400§	22000
PNA+: - Total	720	1600
- T_M enriched	600	1550
- T_M depleted	800	1240
PNA⁻: - Total	6150	63000
- T_M enriched	7700	99500
- T_M depleted	1700	11000

Results concerning a representative experiment out of ten.

*PHA was added at 5 µg/ml
§Cpm/well; Cpm of unstimulated thymocytes have been
subtracted from the values indicated.

Results regarding low cellular concentration (0.5×10^6
ml) experiments clearly indicated that only T_M subset from
PNA⁻ medullary population is able to respons to PHA. By increasing cell concentration to $2.5 \cdot 10^6$/ml the level of stim
ulation increased, and the maximum stimulation occurred ear
lier. The increased blastic trasformation was exhibited
once more by T_M medullary thymocytes.

These data suggested that contact with mitogen alone
by the more mature thymocyte subpopulation was inadequate
for stimulation, and that cells were vigorously stimulated
only in conditioned medium. This conclusion was further sup
ported by the observation that PNA⁻ T_M cells showed mitogenic response only slightly lower than that exhibited by
peripheral blood T cell strongly depleted from macrophages.

Moreover we found that PNA⁻ cells are able to produce significant amount of IL2: culture supernatants from PHA-stimulated PNA⁻ thymocytes exhibited about 1/3 of the growth factor activity displayed by a similar number of PHA⁻ stimulated normal spleen cells or pheripheral lymphocytes.

The proliferative response to PHA at 84 hrs exhibited by the various thymocyte subsets in the presence of exogeneous IL1; IL2 or both are reported in Table II.

TABLE II: Mitogenic response to PHA of thymocyte subsets*

Thymocyte fraction:	None	IL1	IL2	IL1+IL2
Unseparated	3400§	7000	8400	10200
PNA⁺:				
- Total	720	650	1200	1400
- T_M enriched	600	860	1400	1640
- T_M depleted	800	720	1300	1500
PNA⁻:				
- Total	6150	17000	14500	21000
- T_M enriched	7700	24000	19000	26500
- T_M depleted	1700	3300	4800	6600

Results concerning a representative experiment out of ten.

*PHA was added ar 5 µg/ml

Cells: 0.5×10^6/ml

§Cpm/well; Cpm of unstimulated thymocytes have been subtracted from the values indicated.

A pronounced increase of the blastic responses is shown mainly by PNA⁻ cells bearing Fc-IgM receptor. The very poor responses displayed by the PNA⁺, cortical thymo-

cytes can not be significantly enhanced either increasing
cellular density or by adding IL1, IL2 or both in short
term colture (88 hrs) at low cell density.

CONCLUSIONS

From these results the following conclusions can be
drawn:

- The most advanced intrathymic maturative step is attained
by PNA⁻ medullary, T_M cells.
- PNA unagglutinable thymocytes are able to produce significant amounts of IL2.
- IL2 alone can increase the blastic proliferation of
thymocytes but its activity is restricted in short term
culture to medullary compartment.
- The highest mitogenic responses are obtained by the syner
gistic action of IL1 and IL2. One explanation for this
last observation is the possibility that IL1 is essential
for T cell dependent IL2 production in human.In the thymus
like in human pheripheral blood (Smith, et al., 1980) the
mechanism of the lymphoproliferative effect of IL1 produced
by macrophages could be mediated by the stimulation of the
release of T cell growth factor (IL2) by T cell: so that
the magnitude of the resultant T cell proliferation is
dependent upon the quantity of both IL1 and IL2 induced by
lectin stimulation.

REFERENCES

Blyden, G. and Handschumacher, R.E.: Purification and
    properties of Human Lymphocytes Activating
    Factor (LAF). J. Immunol. 118; 1631, 1977.
Gillis, S., Ferm, M.M., Ou, W. and Smith, K.A.:
    T Cell Growth Factor: Parameters of Production and A
    Quantitative Microassay for Activity. J. Immunol., 120
    2027, 1978.

Irlè, C.: Rapid Purification of Peanut Agglutinin by Sialic
    Acid-Less Fetuin-Sepharose Column. J. Immunol.Methods
    17: 1170, 1977.
Mizel, S.B. and Farrar, J.: Revised Nomenclature for Anti
    gen-Nonspecific T-Cell Proliferation and Helper
    Factors. Cell. Immunol. 48: 433, 1979.
Musiani, P., Lauriola, L., Carbone, A., Piantelli, M. and
    Dina, M.A.: Expression of IgM-Fc Receptors by Human
    Thymocytes. In: Aiuti, F. and Wigzell, H., (Editors).
    Thymus, Thymic Hormones and T Lymphocytes. Proceedings
    of the Serono Symposia, Vol. 38° p. 89, Academic Press
    London, 1980.
Musiani, P., Lauriola, L., Carbone, A., Maggiano, N. and
    Piantelli, M.: Lymphocyte Subsets in Human Thymus:
    Expression of IgM-Fc Receptors by Peanut Agglutinin
    Positive and Negative Thymocytes. Thymus, in press.
Reisner, Y., Biniaminov, M., Rosenthal, E., Sharon, N. and
    Ramot, B.: Interaction of Peanut Agglutinin with Nor
    mal Human Lymphocytes and with Leukemic Cells. Proc.
    Natl. Acad. Sci. Usa. 76: 447, 1979.
Smith, K.A., Lachman, L.B., Oppenheim, J.J. and Favata, M.
    F.: The Functional Relationship of the Interleukins.
    J. Exp. Med. 151: 1551, 1980.

B-LYMPHOCYTES DIFFERENTIATION IN
ADULT HUMAN BONE-MARROW

G.C. De Gast, TAE Platts-Mills.

Clinical Research Centre Harrow London,

Division of Immunohaematology,

University Hospital Utrecht.

ABSTRACT

B lymphocytes from adult bone marrow develop IgM surface markers and are stimulatory in the MRL, but are incapable to fully respond to PWM stimulation with proliferation and Ig production. The density of IgM surface markers is lower than that recorded in peripheral blood B cells.

INTRODUCTION

During prenatal development B cell generation and differentiation in man occurs in fetal liver and bone marrow as in the mouse. In adult life it problably occurs only in bone marrow. The aim of this study was to investigate the functional capacity of B lymphocytes from adult human bone marrow in order to obtain evidence of funtional immaturity of these cells. As immuno-globulin (Ig) production is the most clear-cut B cell function, we studied pokeweed mitogen (PWM)-induced Ig production in vitro.

RESULTS AND DISCUSSION

Bone marrow (BM) was obtained from rib section removed during thoracotomy on ten patients (mean age 45 years) with a primary lung tumour. A linear sucrose-serum density gradient was used to fractionate the nucleated bone marrow cells. The pellet fraction which contained only a few lymphocytes, but nearly all the morphological plasma cells showed spontaneous IgM and IgG production. The upper fraction (5-8% sucrose), comprising 82% lymphoid cells (24.2% T cells and 14.0% B cells (SmIg+ve cells) showed no spontaneous Ig production, but in five cases produced Ig when stimulated with pokeweed mitogen (PWM). After T/non T cell separation of this lymphocyte rich (upper) fraction the BM-non T cells produced little or no Ig on their own even when stimulated with PWM. However, these cells produced IgM (mean 0.57 ug/ml) and/or IgG (mean 1.69 ug/ml) when cultured with mitomycin-C treated allogeneic peripheral blood T cell (PB-Tm) and PWM. Parallel cultures of similarly separated PB-non T cells in the presence od PWM and the same PB-Tm produced significantly more Ig (mean IgM 6.02 ug//ml mean IgG 5.33 ug/ml).

In seven preparations from adult human bone marrow (BM) surface IgM positive (SmTgM+ve)cells were detected with anti-IgM coated ox red blood cells (anti-IgM-OxRBC).

On average SmIgM+ve cells in the lymphocyte rich fractions from BM bound fewer anti-IgM-OxRBC than peripheral blood (PB) SmIgM+ve cells.

After isolation on a ficol/metrizoate gradient BM sIgM+ve cells were cultured with mitomycin-C treated PB T cells and pokeweed mitogen (PWM). These cells produced 0.44 ± 052 ug IgM/ml and only 0.10 ± 0.11 IgG/ml. By contrast, PB sIgM+ve cells under similar conditions produced 11.5 ± 10.4 ug IgM/ml and 6.5 ± 7.0 ug IgG/ml. In addition, BM sIgM+ve cells showed very poor PWM induced thymidine incorporation in cultures with PB Tm (mean stimulation index 2.5 ± 2.0) compared to sIgM+ve cells from PB (mean 29.9 ± 25.3). On the other hand, the stimulator capacity of BM sIgM+ve cells in the mixed lymphocyte reaction was similar to that of PB sIgM+ve cells (mean stimulation ratio, BM: 11.1 ± 7.2; PB: 18.9 ± 14.6). The results suggest that B lymphocytes in adult BM develop IgM surface markers and the ability to stimulate in the MLR without becoming fully responsive to PWM for Ig production or proliferation. In addition, these "immature" B cells appear to have less IgM on their surface than PB B cells.

SESSION II

THE THYMIC MICROENVIRONMENT

HUMORAL FUNCTION OF THE THUMAN THYMUS

Robert Oosterom and Louis Kater

Division of Immunopathology

Departments of Internal Medicine and Pathology

University Hospital, Utrecht, The Netherlands

ABSTRACT

Human thymic epithelial conditioned medium (HTECM) increases the reactivity of human and mouse thymocytes to concanavalin A (Con A) and phytohemagglutinin (PHA), and the reactivity of mouse thymocytes after allogeneic stimulation. Target cells for HTECM in subpopulations of mouse thymocytes at various times after hydrocortisone (HC) treatment were investigated. The PHA but not the Con A response of cortisone-resistant thymocytes (T_{cr}, Day 3 after HC) was augmented by HTECM. Twelve days after HC treatment the thymus contained a population of cells (T_{12}) unresponsive to Con A and PHA and unresponsive to HTECM. Between Days 17 and 19 the mitogen response was still very low but HTECM induced a marked increase in mitogen reactivity. After Day 19 the responses gradually returned to normal values. In the presence of T_{cr} T_{12} could be stimulated by mitogens. This response of mixtures of T_{12} and T_{cr} to mitogen was increased by HTECM.

Thymus function decreases at aging. This may be due to changes either in thymocyte population or in thymus microenvironment, both of which were studied. Human thymocyte responsiveness to Con A and PHA increased with age. Thymocytes sensitive to HTECM modulation with Con A as mitogen were found in all age groups. With PHA as mitogen only thymocytes from individuals under the age of 8 years were sensitive to HTECM. Activity of HTECM from cultured thymic epithelial cells grown from individuals of different ages rose to a peak at individuals around 20 years of age and declined afterwards. Involution and lymphodepletion of the thymus with age thus appears to be attended with changes in cellular and epithelial function.

INTRODUCTION

Human thymic epithelial conditioned medium (HTECM), a humoral factor secreted by cultured thymic epithelial cells, enhances the Con A and PHA responsiveness of human and mouse thymocytes (Oosterom et al., 1979), and augments the proliferative and cytotoxic response of mouse thymocytes after stimulation with allogeneic cells; and preincubation of mouse thymocytes with HTECM renders the cells more reactive in in vivo graft-vs-host reactions (Oosterom and Kater, 1980a). These effects are not found with control conditioned media obtained from fibroblast cultures and epithelial cultures from non-lymphoid organs. Target cells for HTECM are found in human and mouse thymocytes and in mouse spleen cells, but not in human peripheral blood lymphocytes and mouse lymph node cells (Oosterom et al., 1979). The thymocytes, used as target cells for HTECM, are obtained from normal thymuses and consist of a heterogeneous population in different stages of maturation. In this paper we describe the effects of HTECM on thymocyte subpopulations obtained from mice several days after hydrocortisone (HC) treatment. With these data we propose the sites of action of HTECM in thymocyte maturation. Additionally we report on the functional changes occurring in the aging human thymus both at the level of thymocytes and of epithelial cells.

MATERIAL AND METHODS

Tissue cultures

Human thymic epithelial cells were cultured in HEPES-buffered RPMI-1640 (H-RPMI) with 20% heatinactivated human AB serum, 2 mM L-glutamine, 100 U/ml penicillin and 100 µg/ml streptomycin (Oosterom et al., 1979; Oosterom and Kater, 1981b). Conditioned media were collected twice a week and filtered before storage at $-20^{o}C$. Conditioned media from cultures of human labial epithelial cells (HLECM) served as controls.

Lymphocyte cultures

Mouse thymocytes were cultured in round bottom microtiter plates in H-RPMI with bicarbonate, glutamine, antibiotics, and 10% AB serum at a density of $2 \times 10^{5}/0.15$ ml/well. Con A (2 µg/well) and PHA 16 µg/well) were added together with HTECM or control conditioned medium in a final dilution of 1:15 to 1:18 resulting in optimal effects on mitogen response (Oosterom et al., 1979). The cells were cultured for two days and labelled with 1 µCi ^{3}H-TdR during the last seven hours. Human thymocytes were cultured at a density of $5 \times 10^{5}/0.15$ ml/well for four days and labelled with ^{3}H-TdR during the last 16 hours. Mitogen concentration used were Con A 2 µg/well and PHA 16 µg/well.

Mice and hydrocortisone treatment

Female Swiss mice aged 6-12 weeks were used. Mice were injected with 2.5 mg of hydrocortisone-acetate (HC) at different times prior to the experiment.

RESULTS

Target cell for HTECM in mouse thymic lymphocyte population

In order to evaluate the thymocyte population affected by HTECM, mice were injected with HC. The effect of HTECM on mitogen responsiveness to thymocytes from mice at various days after HC treatment was studied to investigate its effect on cortisone resistant thymocytes (T_{cr}, Day 3 after HC) and on immature lymphocytes entering the thymus during the repopulation period. As shown in Figs. 1.a. and b. there was a relative increase in reactivity to both Con A and PHA in the first 5 days after HC treatment when the total thymic cell number diminshed. During the subsequent regeneration of the thymus the reactivity to both mitogens decreased and reached a minimum below control values, around Day 12. As can be noted in Fig. 1.a. the effect of HTECM on ^{3}H-TdR incorporation in Con A-stimulated thymocytes was absent at Days 3-5, reached normal levels at Day 7 and was absent again around Day 12. The increase in ^{3}H-TdR incorporation in PHA-stimulated thymocytes caused by HTECM was maximal at Days 3-5 and dropped to zero around Day 12 Fig. 1.b.). The mitogen reactivity of thymocytes and the effect of HTECM reached normal levels at Day 42.

To get a better understanding of the effect of HTECM on the mitogen response of the different thymocyte subpopulations, mixtures of thymocytes 3 days (T_{cr}) and 12 days (T_{12}) after HC were used (Figs. 2.a. and b.). Con A and PHA response increased with increasing numbers of T_{cr}. The effect of HTECM on the Con A response was already seen with 5% T_{cr} and reached its maximum with 20% T_{cr}; no effect was seen with either 100% T_{cr} or 100% T_{12}. The effect of HTECM on the PHA response increased with rising numbers of T_{cr} and was maximal with 100% T_{cr}.

Aging of the human thymus

In a previous study we have found that thymocytes from older donors seemed to respond better to Con A and PHA. To investigate a possible relationship between age of thymusdonor and proliferative response of thymocytes, thymidine incorporation into 5×10^5 stimulated thymocytes from donors of different age groups were compared. The results of TdR incorporation into Con A- and PHA-stimulated cultures according to age groups is shown in Table 1. The PHA response was about six-fold higher than the Con A response. The highest Con A and PHA responses for thymo-

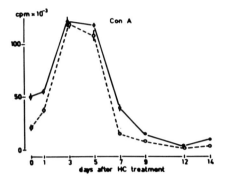 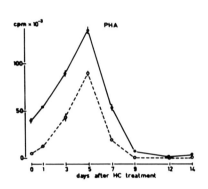

Figure 1

^{3}H-TdR incorporation into Con A (1.a.) or PHA (1.b.) stimulated mouse thymocytes, obtained from mice various days after HC treatment, cultured with
HTECM at a dilution of 1:30 (———) or without conditioned medium (---). Each
point is the mean ± SE of 3 different experiments. Bars are omitted if they
are smaller than the figures.

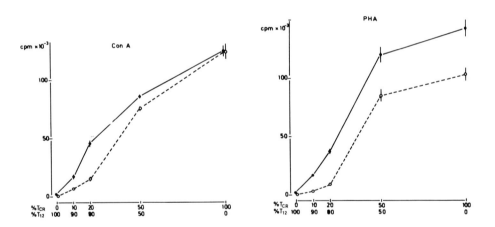

Figure 2

The dotted line represents the ^{3}H-TdR incorporation into mixtures of T_{cr}
and T_{12} stimulated with Con A (2.a.) or PHA (2.b.). The continuous line
shows the H-TdR incorporation when HTECM at a dilution of 1:30 was added.
T_{cr}: thymocytes obtained 3 days after HC treatment; T_{12}: thymocytes obtained 12 days after HC treatment. Each point is the mean ± SE of 3
different experiments.

cytes have been found in age group I, the incorporation was low in age
group II and increased with advancing age.

The Con A response of thymocytes from all donors was enhanced by
HTECM, as was the PHA response of thymocytes from donors in age groups
II (Table 1). No effect was seen on the PHA response of thymocytes
from donors in age group I, III and IV.

The relative activity of HTECM in dilution 1:30 on Con A and PHA
responsiveness of mouse thymocytes is shown in Fig. 3. The activity of
HTECM from normal thymic tissue seemed to be highest at 15-20 years of
age. The same results were obtained with HTECM in dilution 1:15. The
mean activity of HTECM from donors under the age of 30 years was significantly higher ($P < 0.01$) than that from donors above 30 years of
age, for both dilutions tested.

DISCUSSION

Several thymic humoral factors have been described inducing T lymphocyte maturation. Most of these are whole thymic extracts, which makes
it difficult to discriminate between epithelial and lymphocytic factors.
Supernatants from thymic epithelial cultures can be used to ge around
this difficulty. We have shown previously that HTECM enhances the mitogenic response of thymocytes but not of more mature cells, like peripheral blood cells and lymph node cells (Oosterom et al., 1979; Oosterom
and Kater, 1980a).

Target cells for HTECM in the mouse thymus

Target cell subpopulations in the mouse thymus were studied on
several days after HC treatment. Three days after HC treatment the
thymus contains mainly mature, cortisone-resistant thymocytes (T_{cr}).
These cells are comparable with normal spleen cells in their responsiveness to mitogen and sensitivity to HTECM. Twelve days after HC treatment
the thymus contains a mainly immature lymphocyte population, in respect
of mitogen responsiveness as well as based on morphlogy. In cooperation
with dr. S. Kuang Hu and dr. A.L. Goldstein, G. Washington University,
Washington D.C., these observations were extended by measurement of the
enzym terminal deoxynucleotidyl transferase (TdT) content in thymocytes.
A high level of TdT is a marker for immature T cells (Kung et al., 1975).
The TdT level in a pool of T_{12} cells is about four times higher than in
normal thymocytes, and gradually decreases to normal levels between

TABLE 1 - THYMOCYTE RESPONSES TO CON A AND PHA AND THE EFFECT OF HTECM ON
THESE RESPONSES[1]

Group[2]	n	Con A		PHA	
		cpm ± SE	PE[3]	cpm ± SE	PE
I	6	13 784 ± 2 289	1.83	87 931 ± 24 893	1.50
II	16	3 648 ± 482	1.97	18 522 ± 5 014	2.35
III	7	4 603 ± 1 153	2.01	74 333 ± 26 143	1.17
IV	5	8 175 ± 3 074	1.78	57 056 ± 18 946	1.37

[1] Thymocytes were cultured at a concentration of 10×10^5 cells/culture.
[2] Age range: group I, < 6 mo; group II, 6 mo - 6 yr; group III
7 yr - 18 yr; group IV 19 yr - 33 yr.
[3] Potentiating effect (PE): factor by which the response to mitogen is
increased by HTECM.

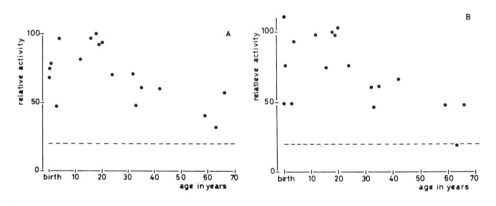

Figure 3
Relative activity of HTECM obtained from epithelial cultures of normal
thymus tissue (●). Panel A, activity of HTECM at a dilution of 1:30 on the
Con A response of mouse thymocytes; Panel B, activity of HTECM at a dilution of 1:30 on the PHA response. Identical results were obtained with
HTECM at a dilution of 1:15. In the dotted line the activity of control
conditioned media are represented.

Days 12 and 19 after HC treatment. When cultured with HTECM during a two day culture period T_{12} cells develop into cells, which are capable to respond to mitogen but only in presence of T_{cr} or lymph node (LN) cells or supernatants from mitogen stimulated LN cells (Oosterom and Kater, 1979). A three day culture period of T_{12} cells with HTECM renders thymocytes directly responsive to mitogen (Oosterom, 1980). Mature lymphocytes or their products do not by themselves induce maturation of immature cells, but act as a second signal after mitogenic (or allogeneic) activation (see next paragraph).

Comparison between mode of action of HTECM and factors from macrophages and lymphocytes

Factors from macrophages and activated lymphocytes have been described that are able to enhance immune reactivity of T lymphocytes. Because presence of macrophages and lymphocytes cannot be totally excluded in thymus tissue cultures, factors of these cell types are discussed here.

Coculturing of thymocytes with peritoneal macrophages increases mitogen responsiveness (Van den Tweel and Walker, 1977). Coculturing of gradient-purified immature thymocytes with thymic macrophages induces phenotypes of mature T lymphocytes (Beller and Unanue, 1978). Therefore it has been proposed that macrophages can regulate thymocyte differentiation. Macrophages produce several factors originally called LAF (lymphocyte activating factor) (Gery et al., 1972).These factors have been recently renamed (Mizel and Farrar, 1979), and are now called Interleukin 1 (IL-1). Amongst other activities LAF has been shown to enhance the mitogen response and MLC reactivity of mouse thymocytes (Oppenheim et al., 1976). LAF exerts its enhancing effect on the mitogen response of LN cells when present from 16 to 24 hours after the start of the cultures (Kierszenbaum and Waksman, 1977a, b). Recently, it has been demonstrated that thymocytes become sensitive to macrophage culture fluid (MCF) after a brief Con A pulse, but the reverse preincubation of thymocytes with MCF does not result in increased Con A responsiveness (Beller and Unanue, 1979). This provides evidence that MCF acts as a second signal after mitogenic activation. The observations on the mode of action of LAF, mentioned above, permit a similar conclusion. Macrophages are present in the thymus and may be present in thymic epithelial cultures, and thus, HTECM may contain LAF. However, our results make such a possibility unlikely for the following reasons: 1) HTECM is hardly mitogenic for thymocytes, while LAF is extremely mitogenic (Gery et al., 1972). 2) Preincubation of thymocytes with HTECM results in increased mitogen response (Oosterom, 1980) and graft-vs-host reaction (Oosterom and Kater, 1980a) in contrast to preincubation with MCF (Beller and Unanue, 1979). 3) HTECM exerts its maximum potentiating effect when present at the start of the culture (Oosterom and Kater, 1981c), while LAF is most effective when present from 16 to 24 hours after initiation of the cultures. 4) Additionally, it is likely that control tissue cultures also contain macrophages, but control conditioned media do not express HTECM activities on thymocytes.

Upon activation mature T lymphocytes produce lymphokines that enable immature T cells to respond to mitogen or alloantigen. Several groups have described lymphokines with such activities: active supernatants (Jacobsson and Blomgren, 1975), costimulator (Paetkau et al., 1976), and T cell growth factor (TCGF) (Smith et al., 1979). The production of costimulator (Mills et al., 1976) and TCGF (Smith et al., 1979) has been proven to be macrophage dependent, but actually they are produced by T lymphocytes (Paetkau et al., 1976; Gillis et al., 1978). Costimulator and mitogen are both required for proliferation (Mills et al., 1976); further it has been shown that TCGF provides the mitogenic stimulus after lectin or antigen binding to the cell membrane (Smith et al., 1979). Referring to the fact that TCGF is the best described lymphocyte factor, TGCF will be used in the further discussion, although these lympocyte factors are now called Interleukin 2 (IL-2) (Mizel and Farrar, 1979). Smith et al. (1979) have postulated the following model for T cell proliferation: 1) Mature T lymphocytes cooperate with adherent cells upon interaction with mitogen or antigen, and TCGF is released. Immature T cells (TCGF-responsive cells) simultaneously acquire the capacity to react to TCGF following mitogen or antigen activation. 2) The proliferative signal is mediated solely by TCGF and mitogen or antigen is no longer necessary. We have shown that, in the presence of T_{cr} or LN cells which are TCGF-producing cells (Gillis et al., 1978) T_{12} cells respond to mitogen; and this response is enhanced by HTECM. Difference in activity between HTECM and TCGF has been substantiated by 1) the absence of TCGF activity in HTECM (Oosterom and Kater, 1980b); 2) the capacity of HTECM to enhance the reactivity of T_{12} cells in the presence of TCGF-producing cells; 3) the observation that TCGF acts as a second signal. From the experiments described herein it appears that TCGF-responsive cells are present in T_{12} cells and that the number of TCGF-responsive cells or their reactivity is increased by HTECM. TCGF-responsive cells have been found in mouse thymus and spleen (Smith et al., 1979) and in nude mouse spleen (Gillis et al., 1979). It may therefore be postulated that immature cell populations contain TCGF-responsive cells and that their number of reactivity increases under the influence of the thymus. Recently it has been shown that rat thymic epithelial supernatant (TES) and TCGF have distinct effects on the generation of cytotoxic T cells by thymocyte subpopulations. PNA^+ thymocytes contain precursor cytotoxic T lymphocytes (CTL) which can be activated in the presence of T helper cells or TCGF. TES induces T_{12} helper cells in PNA^+ thymocytes which in turn help the precursor CTL to develop in effector CTL (Kruisbeek et al., 1980).

Sites of action for HTECM

Based on the data obtained with T_{12} cells and the above described effects of TCGF and LAF, we suggest hypothetical sites of action for HTECM in thymic cell maturation, which are presented in Fig. 4. Prethymic precursor cells (pre-T) migrate from bone marrow to the thymus and differentiate under the influence of the thymus microenvironment to thymocytes ($T_{cortex\ 1}$), which are probably mainly located in the outer cortex. These cells may form the major part of the T_{12} population. When cultured with HTECM during a two day culture period they develop into thymocytes ($T_{cortex\ 2}$), which are capable to respond to mitogen in the presence of TCGF. A prolonged culture of T_{12} with HTECM renders thymocytes directly responsive to mitogen, and therefore resemble medullary thymocytes ($T_{medulla}$). These cells produce TCGF, which in turn allows the cortical thymocytes to proliferate.

The thymus at aging

Human thymocytes can respond to Con A and PHA but the number of cells needed for stimulation is much higher than that of PBL (Oosterom and Kater, 1981a). A remarkable observation is the high proliferative

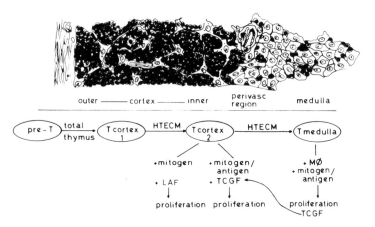

Figure 4
Hypothetical sites of action for HTECM, TCGF and LAF in thymocyte maturation.

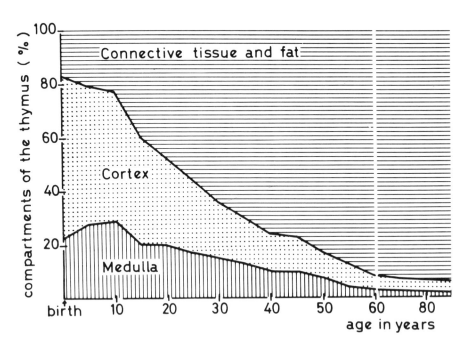

Figure 5
Compartments of the thymus in relation to age, expressed as volume per-
centage of total thymus (data derived from: Boyd, 1936, Baak, 1974;
Simpson et al., 1975; Singh and Singh, 1979)

response of thymocytes from donors under the age of six months (Table 1). The response of these cells to the mitogens tested is higher than that of thymocytes in the other age groups. An explanation for the high proliferative response of thymocytes in age group I may be the fact that we are dealing with a group of highly stressed patients, operated because of cyanosis or rapidly progressive heart failure. This situation does not hold for the other groups of patients who are commonly operated in a stable phase of the disease.

During thymus involution the cortex appears to involute $2\frac{1}{2}$ times faster than the medulla (Singh and Singh, 1979), which results in a relative predominance of the more mature, medullary thymocytes in the thymus of older individuals (Fig. 5). This shift to more mature thymocytes in the aging thymus can explain the increase in mitogen responsiveness and the decline in sensitivity to HTECM at aging. The explanation for a modified thymocyte composition may be an age related decrease in bone marrow thymocyte precursors (Tyan, 1977). It may also be attributed to a diminished thymic function with age, resulting in reduced thymocyte differentation. The following observations in mice support the view that the cause for this diminished cellular immunity in old individuals lies in the thymus itself, rather than in the bone marrow: 1) Bone marrow from old mice give normal immunocompetence in young recipients (Harrison et al., 1977). 2) The involuted thymus is less effective in T cell differentiation (Hirokawa and Makinodan, 1975), which may, at least partly, be related to the diminished secretion of thymic factors.

The activity of HTECM from thymic epithelial cultures established from older individuals is lower than that from younger individuals. Highest activity is found at 15-20 years of age (Fig. 3). This finding corresponds with reports by others on the levels of thymus derived factors in the circulation, like thymopoietin (Lewis et al., 1978), serum thymic factor (Wyermans and Astaldi, 1978), and serum factor (Dardenne et al., 1974). Thus, at least in vitro, thymic factor production by thymic epithelial cells from older individuals is diminished. In all studies on thymus-dependent activity in serum maximum activity has been reported around 20 years, thereafter a decrease was noted. Total thymic mass diminishes with aging (Boyd, 1936), as well as the thymus parenchy-

48

ma (Simpson et al., 1975) and the number of Hassall's corpuscles (Boyd,
1936), which reflects thymic epithelial activity (Kater, 1976). Due to
diminished epithelium levels of thymic factors decrease. Severe thymic
involution has been associated with a decline in circulating thymopoietin activity (Lewis et al., 1978). Further a diminished ability of
aging thymus to reconstitute thymectomized mice has been shown (Hirokawa
and Makinodan, 1975). In our in vitro system the activity of HTECM declines with age as does the activity of thymic dependent factors in serum.
This activity is not correlated with the number of epithelial cells since
all cultures were used near complete confluency. Thus, implying that
also intrinsic changes in the epithelial cells from aging individuals
can contribute to the diminished secretion of thymic factors, resulting
in decline of serum thymic-hormone-like activity with aging.

ACKNOWLEDGMENTS

We thank mr. J.G.N. Geertzema for technical assistance and miss
M. Snellenberg for expert administrative help.

REFERENCES

Baak, J.P.A., 1974: The thymus and sudden infant death syndrome; a
    stereological analysis. Thesis, Amsterdam, The Netherlands.
Beller, D.I. and Unanue, E.R., 1978: Thymic macrophages modulate one
    stage of T cell differentiation in vitro. J. Immunol. 121: 1861.
Beller, D.I. and Unanue, E.R., 1978: Evidence that thymocytes require
    at least two distinct signals to proliferate. J. Immunol. 123:
    2890.
Boyd, E., 1936: Weight of the thymus and its component parts and number
    of Hassall's corpuscles in health and in disease. Am. J. Dis. Child.
    51: 313.
Dardenne, M., Papiernik, M., Bach, J.F. and Stutman, O., 1974: Studies
    on thymus products. III. Epithelial origin of the serum thymic
    factor. Immunology 27: 299.
Gery, I., Gershon, R.K. and Waksman, B.H., 1972: Potentiation of the
    T-lymphocyte response to mitogens. I. The responding cell. J. Exp.
    Med. 136: 128.
Gillis, S., Ferm, M.M., Ou, W. and Smith, K.A., 1978: T cell growth
    factor: parameters of production and a quantitative microassay for
    activity. J. Immunol. 120: 2027.
Gillis, S., Union, N.A., Baker, P.E. and Smith, K.A., 1979: The in
    vitro generation and sustained culture of nude mouse cytolytic T-
    lymphocytes. J. Exp. Med. 149: 1460.
Harrison, D.E., Astle, C.M. and Doubleday, J.W., 1977: Stem cell lines
    from old immunodeficient donors give normal responses in young
    recipients. J. Immunol. 118: 1223.

Hirokawa, K. and Makinodan, T., 1975: Thymus involution: Effect on T cell differentiation. J. Immunol. 114: 1659.

Jacobsson, H. and Blomgren, H., 1975: Evidence of different cell populations in the mouse thymus releasing and responding to mitogenic factor. Scand. J. Immunol. 4: 791.

Kater, L., 1970: Morphological and dynamic aspects of the thymus. Thesis, Utrecht, The Netherlands.

Kierszenbaum, F. and Waksman, B.H., 1977a: Mechanisms of action of lymphocyte activating factor. I. Association of lymphocyte activating factor action with early DNA synthesis in PHA-stimulated lymphocytes. Immunology 33: 663.

Kierszenbaum, F. and Waksman, B.H., 1977b: Kinetics of the potentiation of DNA synthesis by lymphocyte activating factor. In: D.O.Lucas (Editor), Regulatory Mechanisms in Lymphocyte Activation, Academic Press, New York, pp. 704-706.

Kruisbeek, A.M., Zijlstra, J.J. and Kröse, T.J.M., 1980: Distinct effects of T cell growth factors and thymic epithelial factors on the generation of cytotoxic T lymphocytes by thymocyte subpopulations. J. Immunol. 125: 995.

Kung, P.C., Silverstone, A.E., McCaffrey, R.P. and Baltimore, D., 1975: Murine terminal deoxynucleotidyl transferase: cellular distribution and response to cortisone. J. Exp. Med. 141: 855.

Lewis, V.M. Twomey, J.J., Balmear, P., Goldstein, G. and Good, R.A., 1978: Age, thymic involution, and circulating thymic hormone activity. J. Clin. Endocrinol. Metab. 47: 145.

Mills, G., Monticone, V. and Paetkau, V., 1976: The role of macrophages in thymocyte mitogenesis. J. Immunol. 117: 1325.

Mizel, S.B. and Farrar, J.J., 1979: Revised nomenclature for antigen-nonspecific T-cell proliferation and helper factors. Cell. Immunol. 48: 433.

Oosterom, R., 1980: Humoral function of the human thymus. Thesis, Utrecht, The Netherlands.

Oosterom, R. and Kater, L., 1979: Effects of conditioned media of human thymus epithelial cultures on T-lymphocyte functions. Ann. N.Y. Acad. Sci. 332: 113.

Oosterom, R. and Kater, L., 1980a: Effect of human thymic epithelial conditioned medium on in vitro and in vivo alloantigen-induced lymphocyte activation in het mouse. Clin. Immunol. Immunopathol. 17: 173.

Oosterom, R. and Kater, L., 1980b: Target cell subpopulations for human thymic epithelial conditioned medium in the mouse thymus. Clin. Immunol. Immunopathol. 17: 183.

Oosterom, R. and Kater, L., 1981a: The thymus in the aging individual. I. Mitogen responsiveness of human thymocytes. Clin. Immunol. Immunopathol.: in press.

Oosterom, R. and Kater, L., 1981b: The thymus in the aging individual. II. Thymic epithelial function in vitro in aging and in thymus pathology. Clin. Immunol. Immunopathol.: in press.

Oosterom, R. and Kater, L., 1981c: Studies on the mechanism of action of human thymic epithelial conditoned medium on mouse thymocytes. Evidence for induction of immune competence. Immunopharmacol.: in press.

Oosterom, R., Kater, L. and Oosterom, J., 1979: Effects of human thymic
    epithelial conditioned medium on mitogen responsiveness of human
    and mouse lymphocytes. Clin. Immunol. Immunopathol. 12: 460.
Oppenheim, J.J., Shneyour, A. and Kook, A.I., 1976: Enhancement of DNA
    synthesis and cAMP content of mouse thymocytes by mediator(s)
    derived from adherent cells. J. Immunol. 116: 1466.
Paetkau, V., Mills, G., Gerhart, S. and Monticone, V., 1976: Prolifer-
    ation of murine thymic lymphocytes in vitro is mediated by the
    concanavalin A-induced release of a lymphokine (costimulator).
    J. Immunol. 117: 1320.
Simpson, J.G., Gray, E.S. and Beck, J.S., 1975: Age involution in the
    normal human adult thymus. Clin. Exp. Immunol. 19: 261.
Singh, J. and Singh, A.K., 1979: Age-related changes in human thymus.
    Clin. Exp. Immunol. 37: 507.
Smith, K.A., Gillis, S., Baker, P.E., McKenzie, D. and Ruscetti, F.W.,
    1979: T-cell growth factor-mediated T-cell proliferation. Ann. N.Y.
    Acad. Sci. 332: 423.
Tyan, M.L., 1977: Age-related decrease in mouse T cell progenitors.
    J. Immunol. 118: 846.
Van den Tweel, J.G. and Walker, W.S., 1977: Macrophage-induced thymic
    lymphocyte maturation. Immunology 33: 817.
Wyermans, P. and Astaldi, A., 1978: Effect of aging on thymus-dependent
    serum factor(s). Neth. J. Gerontol. 9: 216.

ULTRASTRUCTURAL INVESTIGATION OF THE LYMPHO-EPITHELIAL AND THE LYMPHO-MESENCHYMAL INTERACTIONS IN THE ONTOGENY OF THE HUMAN THYMUS

B. von Gaudecker and H. K. Müller-Hermelink

Anatomisches Institut der Universität Kiel, Haus N 10 Olshausenstraße, D-2300 Kiel und Abteilung Allgemeine Pathologie und Pathologische Anatomie der Universität Hospitalstraße 42, D-2300 Kiel.

ABSTRACT

The cytological differentiation of human fetal thymocytes has been investigated in relation to the maturation of stationary epithelial and mesenchymal cells and to the development of specific functional cell markers: The thymus primordium in fetuses of the 12th gestational week (GW) contains exclusively precursor-type thymocytes characterized by an irregular convoluted nucleus, a strong focal acid phosphatase activity and simultaneously present sheep-red-blood-cell- and complement-receptors on the cell surface, which can be demonstrated by mixed rosettes. During the 14th GW the cortex and the medulla begin to differentiate. In correlation with this differentiation, the amount of mixed rosette-formation by the precursor-type thymocytes is decreasing, and the amounts of differentiated cortical and medullary thymocytes, which exclusively form rosettes with sheep-red-blood-cells, are increasing. Concurrently, the differentiation of cortical and medullary epithelial cells and the invasion of precursors of interdigitating cells into the thymus medulla can be observed. The interaction of these developing stationary cells with the different lymphoid cells in the fetal human thymus is discussed.

Acknowledgments: This investigation was supported by a grant from the Deutsche Forschungsgemeinschaft and by the Sonderforschungsbereich 111. The authors appreciate the contribution of human fetal material from Dr. von Hollweg and Dr. Körner from the hospital Heidberg c.o. Hamburg, and the excelent technical assistence of Mrs. O.M. Bracker, Mrs. I. Knauer, Mrs. R. Köpke, Mrs. F. Müller, Mrs. H. Siebke and Mrs. H. Waluk.

INTRODUCTION

Cytological studies of acute lymphoblastic leucemias of the T-type revealed a very typical cell type which is characterized by an irregular convoluted nucleus, a strong focal acid phosphatase activity and the presence of sheep-red-blood-cell- and Complement-receptors at the cell surface. Similar cells have been found by our group in the early ontogenesis of the human thymus.

This study has been undertaken in order to characterize the ultrastructural features of early thymic precursor cells, and to correlate their appearance with the maturation of stationary cells and the development of the thymus cortex and the medulla.

The cytological differentiation of the thymocytes shall be dicussed in relation to the acquisition of specific functional cell markers.

MATERIALS AND METHODS

Thymuses from approximately 50 human fetuses were investigated by light- and electron microscopy. The age of the fetuses was calculated from the crown-heal-length and ranged from the 8th to the 28th week of gestation. For methodical details see von Gaudecker and Müller-Hermelink (1980). The histochemical demonstration of acid phosphatase and non-specific esterase as well as the formation of rosettes with sheep erythrocytes and chicken erythrocytes coated with antibody and complement were performed according to Stein and Müller-Hermelink (1976).

RESULTS

The earliest thymic primordium consists entirely of epithelial cells. Later, approximately during the 9th gestational week, it becomes invaded by haemopoietic stem cells.

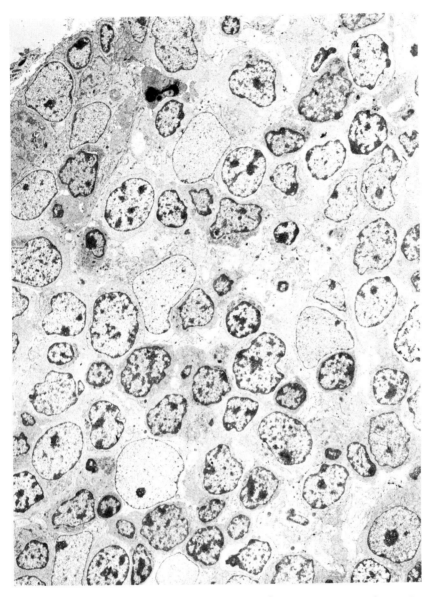

Fig. 1: Human thymus C.H.-length: 8.5 cm, approximately the
12th gestational week. The lymphatic precursor cells have
irregularely outlined nuclei which show a rather finely
distributed heterochromatin pattern. Large electron lucent
nuclei belong to epithelial cells and lymphoblastic cells.

x 7800.

In fetuses of approximately the 12th gestational week
the light microscopical aspect of the thymus practically is
converted. The peripheral areas stain more faintly than the
center of the organ. This impression is caused by a higher
concentration of medium-sized lymphoid precursor cells in
the central part. The more faintly stained aspect of the
periphery is caused by weakly stained large nuclei which
belong to lymphoblastic cells and epithelial cells.

In electron micrographs it becomes obvious that the
lymphatic cells have irregularely outlined nuclei of different sizes which show a rather finely distributed heterochromatin pattern (Fig. 1). These cytological features may
be interpreted as a sign of immaturity.

These immature precursor type lymphocytes of early fetal thymuses comprise polyribosomes, mitochondria and
single flattened cysternae of rough endoplasmic reticulum
in the rather broad cytoplasmic rim (Fig. 2a). The well
developed Golgi field may contain some small darkly stained
granules probably of lysosomal nature.

Between the 14th and 17th week of gestation the cortical
and medullary differentiation is completed. The dark appearance of the cortex is caused by tightly packed small thymocytes.

In fetuses of the 17th gestational week the thymic
cortex is completely differentiated. Small cortical thymocytes show the same shape as in the postnatal thymus (Fig.2b).
They have a rounded or ovoide nucleus. Clumps of hetero-
chromatic material are disposed along the nuclear membrane
and in the nucleoplasm. The rim of scanty cytoplasm contains
free ribosomes, some mitochondria and rare small granules.
These small thymocytes of the cortex have smooth surface membranes which lie closely together without interdigitations.

55

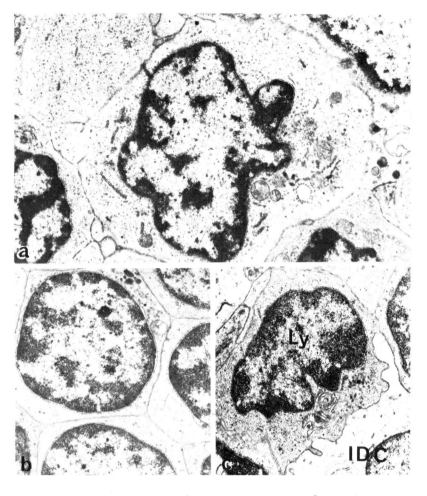

Fig. 2: Human thymus. a): C.H.-length = 8.5 cm, approximately
the 12th gestational week. b) and c): C.H.-length 18 cm
approximately the 17th gestational week.
a) Immature precursor type thymocyte with a irregularely outlined nucleus and a rather broad cytoplasmic rim containing
polyribosomes, mitochondria, single flattened cysternae of
rough endoplasmatic reticulum and a well developed Golgi
field with some darkly stained granules.
b) Small cortical thymocytes with rounded nuclei. Clumps of
heterochromatin material are disposed along the nuclear
membrane and in the nucleoplasm. The smooth surface plasma
membranes lie closely together without interdigitations.
c) Medullary small thymocyte (Ly) in close contact with the
cytoplasm of an interdigitating cell (IDC). Note the bluntly
lobulated nucleus and the small aggregation of lysosomal
structures near the Golgi field.
a) b) c) : x 12 000.

Large lymphoblastic cells with finely dispersed chromatin in their nuclei are found predominantly near the surface
of the organ. Their broad cytoplasmic rim contains free ribosomes mainly as polysomes, mitochondria, some long flattened cysternae of the rough endoplasmic reticulum and a well
developed Golgi region oposite to a nuclear indentation.

The epithelial cells of the cortex have a lightly stained cytoplasm with rare tonofilaments and may contain secretion granules. They send blunt cytoplasmic projections between the lymphoid cells and develop a continous basal la-
mina along the outer surface of the thymus.

Epithelial cells of the medulla develop a different
structure than those in the cortex. Characteristic differences between cortical and medullary epithelial cells may be
seen in fetuses of the 14th gestational week. The medullary
epithelial cells have long, slender processes, and their
cytoplasm is rather darkly stained due to the presence of
abundant tonofilaments. They are associated with the base-
ment membranes, which are composed of a fine filamentous
material.

Beside the epithelial cells, a second stationary cell
type of mesenchymal origin is established in the medulla.
The mesenchymal precursor cells enter the organ by dia-
pedesis and differentiate into interdigitating cells. Their
nuclei are irregularly shaped and have a very loosely
arranged chromatin exept for a characteristic small rim of
heterochromatin along the inner surface of the nuclear
envelope. The lightly stained cytoplasmic projections get
into an intimate contact with medullary small thymocytes
which show in this fetal stage of the 17th gestational week
the morphological features of peripheral T-cells (Fig. 2 c).
Their structure clearly differs from cortical small thymocytes by having a bluntly lobulated nucleus, a well developed
Golgi complex and a small aggregation of lysosomal structures.

TABLE 1

		Fetal stages (gestation weeks)			
		12	14	16	20
Morphological data	Cortex and Medulla	not differentiated	begins to differentiate	fully differentiated	
	Immature (precursor-type) thymocytes	+ + + +	+ + +	+ +	n.t.
	Cortical thymocytes		+ +	+ + +	fully differentiated
	Medullary thymocytes		+ +	+ + +	fully differentiated
	Differences in cortical and medullary epithelial cells	+ +	+ + +	fully differentiated	
	Interdigitating cells in the thymic medulla	Precursors invade the organ	immature	fully differentiated	
Functional data [*]	EAC-rosettes	30%-54%		65%	27%
	E-AET-rosettes	60%		83%	92%
	Mixed rosettes (CH-EAC + EN)	26%-31%		21%	9%
	Focal acP-reactivity	86%-98%		21%	5%
	Focal nonspecific esterase-reactivity	–		+ +	+ + +

Abbreviations

EAC = Erythrocytes coated with antibodies and complement, E-AET = sheep erythrocytes treated with AET, CH-EAC = chicken erythrocytes coated with antibody and complement, EN = sheep erythrocytes treated with neuraminidase, acP = acid phosphatase.

[*] H. Stein and H.K. Müller-Hermelink, Brit. J. Haematol. 36, 225-230 (1977)

Their irregular cytoplasmic protrusions interdigitate with the I.D.C.-s.

CONCLUSIONS

Table 1 summarizes our morphological results and connects them with functional observations from STEIN and MÜLLER-HERMELINK, who could show that lymphocytes isolated from early human fetal thymuses are characterized by con-

voluted nuclei and a strong focal acid phosphatase reactivity in the Golgi field. Simultonously, they bear surface
receptors for complement and sheep red blood cells.

In the early thymus primordium of the 12th gestational
week, we find immature precursor-type thymocytes with an
identical shape. For the same time of ontogeny, the highest
percentages of mixed rosettes could be demonstrated by
STEIN and MÜLLER-HERMELINK!

During the following gestational weeks the amount of
immature thymocytes decreases and becomes replaced by
differentiated cortical and medullary small thymocytes. At
the same time the percentages of EAC-rosettes and mixed
rosettes are decreasing while a considerable increase of
rosettes with sheep erythrocytes is observed. Both, the
morphological and functional results demonstrate the maturation of the lymphoid organization in the fetal thymus.

Before and concurrently with the formation of the
typical "lymphoid defined" structure, the differentiation
of epithelial cells and the invasion of mesenchymal cells
into the thymic medulla occurs which there develope into
I.D.C.-s.

These stationary cells in the thymic cortex and medulla,
provide different microecologies and give a structural basis
for the explanation of the occurence of different types of
lymphoid cells in the cortex and the medulla beginning with
the 14. gestational week.

REFERENCES

Gaudecker, von B. and Müller-Hermelink, H.K.: Ontogeny and
    organization of the stationary non-lymphoid cells in
    the human thymus.
    Cell Tissue Res. 207, 287-306, 1980.
Stein, H. and Müller-Hermelink, H.K.: Simultaneous presence
    for complement and sheep red blood cells on human
    fetal thymocytes.
    British Journal of Haematology 36, 225-230, 1977.

SUPPRESSION OF THE ANTIBODY RESPONSE INDUCED BY MODIFIED SELF
IS PREVENTED BY ADULT THYMECTOMY. RESTORATIVE EFFECT OF
FACTEUR THYMIQUE SERIQUE

B. Grouix[+], D. Erard[+], J. Charreire[*] and P. Galanaud[+]
+ INSERM U 131, 32 rue des Carnets, 92140 Clamart
* INSERM U 25, Hôpital Necker, Paris, France

ABSTRACT

The I.V. injection of trinitrophenyl-conjugated isogeneic spleen
cells (TNP-S.C.) induces a specific suppression of the ability of mice
to respond to the T-independent antigen DNP-Ficoll. This form of
tolerance could not be induced in adult thymectomized (ATX) mice
6 weeks after thymectomy. Treatment of ATX mice with a synthetic
analogue of thymic serum factor (FTS) 7-9 weeks after thymectomy
restores their susceptibility to TNP-S.C.-induced suppression.

INTRODUCTION

The injection of a hapten coupled to syngeneic lymphocytes
constitutes a potent method to suppress the immune response to this
hapten (Miller et al., 1976, Weinberger et al., 1979, Scott, 1978).
Borel et al. (1980) recently shown that this form of suppression could
no more be induced in adult thymectomized (ATX) mice. This work was
designed to better define the role of the thymus in this form of
tolerance, namely whether the hapten-specific suppressor cell (or
its precursor) was dependent on the hormonal influence of the thymus.
We used a synthetic analogue of Facteur Thymique Sérique (Pleau et al.,
1979) (FTS) to answer this question.

MATERIALS AND METHODS

We used 3 to 8 weeks old male Balb/c or CBA mice, obtained from
Charles River (France) and from Chester Beatty Institute (London)
respectively. They were thymectomized at the age of 3 to 4 weeks (ATX).
The hapten-specific suppression was induced by the I.V. injection of

$10'$ trinitrophenyl (TNP) conjugated syngeneic spleen cells (TNP-S.C.)
on two consecutive days (day 0 and day 1). The preparation of TNP-S.C.
was performed according to Scott and Long (1976). Control mice received
the same amount of unconjugated spleen cells (S.C.). The antigenic
challenge took place on day 7, using 10 ug of DNP-Ficoll (a gift of
R. Huchet, Villejuif, France) or sheep red blood cells (SRBC) as a
specificity control in some experiments. The anti-TNP response was
measured 4-5 days later by the haemolytic plaque assay (Jerne et al.
1963). The results were expressed as the number of plaque forming cells
(PFC)/10^6 cells (mean $\pm$ s.e.m. of 4-5 mice in one experiment or of
different experiments, as indicated). The treatment by FTS was
performed as fellows : mice received I.P. 1 ng of FTS on days -2, -1,
0, +1, +4, +5 and +6 of the injection of TNP-S.C. Control groups were
injected with saline. We used a long lived synthetic analogue of FTS
$(D-Ala^6)$ FTS, a gift of M. Dardenne.

RESULTS

Mice treated with TNP-S.C. displayed a markedly depressed response
to the T-independent antigen DNP-Ficoll (see later). This suppression
was strictly antigen specific as shown by their normal response to
SRBC (results not shown). In 4 experiments we shown that 6 weeks after
ATX this suppression could no more be obtained (table 1) (p   0.01 by
the student's test). In order to test the restorative effect of FTS
mice were left untreated for 7-9 weeks after ATX. They were then
treated with FTS (or saline) and TNP-S.C. (or S.C.) as described in
materials and methods. In the intact animals, TNP-S.C. suppressed the
anti-TNP response by 37% in saline-treated animals and by 55% in FTS-
treated animals. In ATX mice the anti-TNP response was virtually
unaffected (9% suppression) in saline-treated mice and suppressed by
48% in FTS-treated mice.

CONCLUSION

These results confirm that the suppression of B cell response by
hapten-modified spleen cells is a T-dependent phenomenon (Borel et al.
1980, Jandinski et al. 1979, Braley-Mullen, 1980) although a direct
suppression of the B cell response has been proposed (Ramos et al. 1980)

Moreover we observed that T cells from TNP-S.C.-treated mice suppress
the in vitro antibody response of normal mouse spleen cells, as
compared to T cells from S.C.-treated animals (Grouix et al.,
submitted for publication). We here show that the suppressor T cells
involved in this form of tolerance are short-lived T cells, which
fits with the demonstration of Jandinski and Scott that they bear
the Ly 1 and the Ly 23 antigens (1979). Our present results indicate
that this cell (or its precursors) are dependent on the hormonal
influence of the thymus. Thus FTS is able to restore several of the
immune functions affected after ATX : optimal cytotoxic T cell
response (Bach, 1977) and contact sensitivity (Erard et al. 1979) as
well as the suppression induced by modified self (this work). As the
mechanism of the latter may be relevant to that of tolerance to self,
this should be considered when evaluating the possibilities of
immunomanipulation in the immunopathological situations where a thymic
dysfunction is present.

TABLE 1 - ATX MICE ARE NO MORE SUPPRESSED BY TNP-S.C.

I.V. pretreatment		anti-TNP response in	
		controls	ATX
S.C.	:	668 + 26	714 + 57
TNP-S.C.	:	350 + 59	701 + 58

REFERENCES

Bach, M.A., 1977. Lymphocyte mediated cytotoxicity : effect of ageing,
     adult thymectomy and thymic factor. J. Immunol., 119: 641.
Borel, Y., Kilham, L., Kurtz, S.E. and Reinisch, C.L., 1980. Dichotomy
     between the induction of suppressor cells and immunologic
     tolerance by adult thymectomy. J. exp. Med., 151: 743.
Braley-Mullen, H., 1980. Suppression of antibody response to type III
     pneumococcal polysaccharide with antigen coupled to syngeneic
     lymphoid cells. Cell. Immunol., 52: 132.

Erard, D., Charreire, J., Auffredou, M.T., Galanaud, P. and Bach, J.F., 1979. Regulation of contact sensitivity to DNFB in the mouse : effects of adult thymectomy and thymic factor. J. Immunol., 123: 1573.

Jandinski, J.J. and Scott, D.W., 1979. Role of self carriers in the immune response and tolerance. IV. Active T cell suppression in the maintenance of B cell tolerance to a "T-independent" antigen. J. Immunol., 123: 2447.

Jerne, N.K. and Nordin, A.A., 1963. Plaque formation in agar by single antibody producing cells. Science, 140: 405.

Miller, S.E. and Claman, H.N., 1976. The induction of hapten specific T cell tolerance by using hapten-modified lymphoid cells. I. Characteristics of tolerance induction. J. Immunol., 117: 1519.

Pleau, J.M., Dardenne, M., Blanot, D., Bricas, E. and Bach, J.F., 1979. Antagonist analogues of serum thymic factor (FTS) interacting with the FTS cellular receptor. Immunol. Letters, 1: 179.

Scott, D.W. and Long, C.A., 1976. Role of self-carriers in the immune response and tolerance. I. B-cell unresponsiviness and cytotoxic T-cell immunity induced by haptenated syngeneic lymphoid cells. J. exp. Med., 144: 1369.

Scott, D.W., 1978. Role of self carriers in the immune response and tolerance. III. B cell tolerance induced by hapten-modified-self involves both active T cell mediated suppression and direct blockade. Cell. Immunol., 37: 327.

Weinberger, J.Z., Germain, R.N., J.U., S.T., Greene, M.I., Benacerraf, B. and Dorf, M.E., 1979. Hapten-specific T cell responses to 4-hydroxy-3-nitrophenyl acetyl. II. Demonstration of idiotypic determinants on suppressor T cells. J. exp. Med., 150: 761.

EFFECT OF ADENOSINE ON NON-HISTONE CHROMATIN PROTEINS OF THYMOCYTES

A. Facchini[*], C.J.M. Leupers[+], L. Cocco[*], G.C.B. Astaldi[+], A.R. Mariani[*],
F.A. Manzoli[*] and A. Astaldi[+]

[*]Istituto di Anatomia Umana Normale, Facoltà di Medicina,
Università di Bologna, Italy

[+]Central Laboratory of the Netherlands Red Cross Blood Transfusion
Service and Laboratory for Experimental and Clinical Immunology,
University of Amsterdam, Amsterdam, The Netherlands

ABSTRACT

The effect of adenosine on the synthesis and on the phosphorylation of
nuclear proteins of thymocytes was investigated after 15 to 240 min of culture. Adenosine was found to induce a rapid increase in the synthesis and
in the phosphorylation of nuclear proteins, especially in the group of non-
histone chromatin proteins. These data suggest that adenosine acts on the
synthesis of phosphorylated non-histone chromatin proteins and may, in this
way, control DNA-template activity.

INTRODUCTION

Previously, we reported that normal human serum contains a thymus-
dependent factor (SF) capable of increasing cAMP in thymocytes and of inducing immunological maturation of thymocytes (Astaldi, A. et al., 1976;
Facchini, et al., 1979; Astaldi, G.C.B. et al., 1980a). SF was purified
and found to be chemically indistinguishable from adenosine (Astaldi, A.
et al., 1980a; Astaldi, A. et al., 1981).

Thus, we investigated whether adenosine (used at the concentrations
found in SF) could also act at the nuclear level of thymocytes. Adenosine
was found to induce mainly synthesis and phosphorylation of non-histone
chromatin proteins (NHCP) in thymocytes.

MATERIALS AND METHODS

Materials and methods have been reported in detail elsewhere (Facchini
et al., 1979). In brief, thymocytes obtained from C57BL/6J mice were exposed to adenosine (10^{-6} M) for 15 to 240 min at 37°C. Nuclear proteins were
isolated after cell fractionation and isolation of chromatin fractions.
Phosphorylate-NHCP (P-NHCP) were obtained by the method of Kleinsmith and

Kish (1975).

Electrophoretic analysis of nuclear proteins, incorporation of ^{3}H-leucine and of ^{32}P-orthophosphate in nuclear proteins were performed as reported (Facchini, et al., 1979).

RESULTS

Table 1 shows the effect of adenosine on the incorporation of ^{3}H-leucine into protein fractions of thymocytes after 30 min incubation.

TABLE 1 - EFFECT OF ADENOSINE ON THE INCORPORATION OF ^{3}H-LEUCINE INTO PRO-
TEIN FRACTIONS OF THYMOCYTES[a]

Substances added	^{3}H-leucine (dpm x 10^{-5}) incorporated per milligram of:				
	Total cell protein	Chromatin	P-NHCP	Histones	R-NHCP
Control	3.0	3.3	14.9	1.7	0.4
Adenosine (10^{-6}M)	6.3	10.1	21.2	2.0	0.6

[a]Each value is the mean of four protein extractions.

At the chromatin level, adenosine induced a marked increase of incorporated radioactivity. When the distribution of radioactivity in the various nuclear proteins (phosphorylated non-histone chromatin proteins (P-NHCP), histones, and residual non-histone chromatin proteins (R-NHCP)) is compared, it is evident that the incorporation of ^{3}H-leucine was especially located in the P-NHCP, which represents only a small amount (about 8%) of the total nuclear proteins. Adenosine induced a high incorporation of ^{3}H-leucine into the P-NHCP as early as after 15 min of culture (not shown). At the level of histones, which represent the highest amount of protein recovered from the chromatin (about 40%), adenosine also induced an increase of incorporation of ^{3}H-leucine, but the specific radioactivity was about one-tenth of that found in the P-NHCP fraction. The incorporation of ^{3}H-leucine into the R-NHCP fraction appeared to be less than 3% of that found in the P-NHCP fraction. Because cycloheximide, a specific inhibitor of protein synthesis, fully prevented the increase in the incorporation of leucine by thymocytes exposed to adenosine, we concluded that adenosine stimulates protein synthesis rather than leucine transport in thymocytes.

Table 2 shows the effect of adenosine on the incorporation of ^{32}P into protein fractions of thymocytes after 30 min of culture. Adenosine induced a marked incorporation of ^{32}P in the total proteins. A similar factor of increase was found to be induced at the chromatin level. When the distribution of radioactivity in the various nuclear fractions is compared, it is evident that the influence of adenosine on the incorporation of ^{32}P was especially marked in the P-NHCP, in analogy with the findings on incorporation of ^{3}H-leucine. Cycloheximide reduced the incorporation of ^{32}P induced by adenosine into proteins of about 50%, indicating that part of the ^{32}P incorporation is due to protein phosphorylation and part is due to the increased protein synthesis. Indomethacin, an inhibitor of cyclic AMP-dependent protein kinase (Kantor and Hampton, 1978), reduced to about 30% the incorporation of ^{32}P induced by adenosine into total thymocyte proteins, further indicating that part of the ^{32}P incorporation reflects protein phosphorylation due to protein kinase activity.

TABLE 2 - EFFECT OF ADENOSINE ON THE INCORPORATION OF ^{32}P INTO PROTEIN FRACTIONS OF THYMOCYTES[a]

Substances added	^{32}P (dpm x 10^{-5}) incorporated per milligram of:				
	Total cell protein	Chromatin	P-NHCP	Histones	R-NHCP
Control	3.6	2.9	0.3	0.2	0.01
Adenosine (10^{-6}M)	7.6	6.9	1.3	0.2	0.04

[a]Each value is the mean of four protein extractions.

Electrophoretic patterns in polyacrylamide gels of the P-NHCP fractions, extracted from the chromatin of the cells stimulated with adenosine, showed that proteins with molecular weights greater than 5×10^4 were synthesized to a larger extent as compared with synthesis in unstimulated cells.

CONCLUSIONS

We concluded that adenosine selectively stimulates synthesis and phosphorylation of high molecular-weight NHCP, as previously found for SF (Facchini, et al., 1979). Since no substantial changes were observed at the histone level, these findings are compatible with DNA transcription and RNA translation. Similarly, polypeptide hormones, such as insulin, prolactin, and chorionic gonadotrophin, as well as steroids (Jungmann and Schweppe, 1972; Spelberg, 1974; Turkington and Riddle, 1969) exert an action on nuclear protein phosphorylation of specific target cells.

In conclusion, the binding of adenosine to thymocytes stimulates adenylate cyclase with a subsequent rise in intracellular cyclic AMP levels; most likely, the increase in cyclic AMP leads to stimulation of protein kinases, since it is known that cyclic AMP regulates the activity of these enzymes (Kuo and Greengard, 1970; Walsh, et al., 1968); protein kinases are, in turn, responsible for the phosphorylation and synthesis of nuclear proteins. The P-NHCP would then be responsible for gene activation (Stein, et al., 1976), which would result in the phenotypic expression of genetic information.

These findings, taken together with the observation that adenosine (at the micromolar level) induces T-cell maturation (Astaldi, A., et al., 1980a; Astaldi, A. et al., 1981) and with the effects previously reported for SF (Astaldi, A. et al., 1980b), suggest that adenosine might be one of the physiological substances modulatory of the immune system.

REFERENCES

Astaldi, A., Astaldi, G.C.B., Schellekens, P.Th.A. and Eijsvoogel, V.P.: Thymic factor in human sera demonstrable by a cyclic AMP assay. Nature 260: 713-715, 1976.

Astaldi, A., Astaldi, G.C.B., Leupers, C.J.M., Brühl, P.C., Bruin, H.G. de, Wijermans, P. and Eijsvoogel, V.P.: The thymus-dependent human serum factor SF. Workshop "Factors of T-cell differentiation", IV. Intern. Congr. Immunol., Paris, 1980a.

Astaldi, A., Astaldi, G.C.B., Wijermans, P., Facchini, A., Bemmel, T. van, Leupers, C.J.M., Schellekens, P.Th.A. and Eijsvoogel, V.P.: In: Polypeptide Hormones. Eds. R.F. Beers Jr. and E.G. Bassett, pp. 501-511 (Raven Press, New York 1980b).

Astaldi, A., Bemmel, T. van, Astaldi, G.C.B., Leupers, C.J.M., Mourik, J.A. van, Hamers, M.N., Loos, J.A., Schellekens, P.Th.A. and Eijsvoogel, V.P.: The thymus-dependent human serum factor SF is adenosine. Submitted for publication, 1981.

Astaldi, G.C.B., Astaldi, A., Wijermans, P., Schellekens, P.Th.A. and Eijsvoogel, V.P.: A thymus-dependent serum factor induces maturation of thymocytes as evaluated by graft-versus-host reaction. Cell. Immunol. 49: 202-207, 1980.

Facchini, A., Astaldi, G.C.B., Cocco, L., Wijermans, P., Manzoli, F.A. and Astaldi, A.: Early events in thymocyte activation. II. Changes in non-histone chromatin proteins induced by a thymus-dependent human serum factor. J. Immunol. 123: 1577-1585, 1979.

Jungmann, R.A. and Schweppe, J.S.: Mechanism of action of gonadotrophin. I. Evidence for gonadotrophin-induced modifications of ovarian nuclear basic and acidic protein biosynthesis, phosphorylation and acetylation. J. Biol. Chem. 247: 5535-5542, 1972.

Kantor, H.S. and Hampton, M.: Indomethacin in submicromolar concentrations inhibits cyclic AMP-dependent protein kinase. Nature 276: 841-842, 1978.

Kleinsmith, L.J. and Kish, V.M.: Methods for analysis of phosphorylated acidic chromatin protein interaction with DNA. In: Methods in Enzymology Vol. 40, Part E:177. Editors L. Grossman and K. Moldave. (Academic Press, New York 1975).

Kuo, J.F. and Greengard, P.: Cyclic nucleotide-dependent protein kinases. VI. Isolation and partial purification of a protein kinase activated

by guanosine 3',5'-monophosphate. J. Biol. Chem. 245: 2493-2498,
   1970.
Spelberg, C.T.: The role of nuclear acidic proteins in binding steroid
   hormones. In: Acidic Proteins of the Nucleus. Editors I.L. Cameron
   and J.R. Jeter Jr., pp. 247-272. (Academic Press, New York 1974).
Stein, G.S., Stein, J.L., Kleinsmith, L.J., Thompson, J.A., Park, W.D. and
   Jansing, R.L.: Role of nonhistone chromosomal proteins in the regula-
   tion of histone gene expression. Cancer Res. 36: 4307-4318, 1976.
Turkington, R.W. and Riddle, M.: Hormone-dependent phosphorylation of nu-
   clear proteins during mammary gland differentiation in vitro. J.
   Biol. Chem. 244: 6040-6046, 1969.
Walsh, D.A., Perkins, J.P. and Krebs, E.G.: An adenosine 3',5'-monophos-
   phate-dependent protein kinase from rabbit skeletal muscle. J. Biol.
   Chem. 243: 3763-3774, 1968.

SESSION III

LYMPHOCYTE DISFUNCTIONS IN AGEING: EXPERIMENTAL APPROACH.

EXPERIMENTAL IMMUNOGERONTOLOGY: A PERSPECTIVE

Diego Segre
Department of Veterinary Pathobiology
University of Illinois
Urbana, Illinois 61801, USA

In these brief opening remarks I do not intend to summarize for you the past accomplishments of immunogerontology. To do so would be presumptous on my part, since most of you in the audience are active in the field and are quite familiar with the relevant literature. Rather, I will try to put experimental immunogerontology in a broader gerontological perspective. To do so I shall ask, and attempt to answer, a number of questions. Both questions and answers will perforce reflect my personal biases. However, they may stimulate you in the audience to subject what I will say to critical examination. This, I hope, will be useful to both you and me.

Does the immune system play a role in aging? This is perhaps the most fundamental question.

During the first, phenomenological phase of immunogerontology, it has been well established that the immune potential declines with advancing age in all mammalian species that have been tested (Makinodan and Kay, 1980). All aspects of the immune response are affected by age, including both humoral and cellular responses and extending to some aspects of natural resistance, such as NK cells (Kiessling and Haller, 1978). Acquired immunologic tolerance, which may be regarded as the counterpart of acquired immunity, is also affected by age, as shown by experiments in which more tolerogen was required to induce tolerance in aged mice than in young-adult mice (McIntosh and Segre, 1976; DeKruyff et al., 1980). In addition, autoimmune phenomena and immunodeficiencies become more frequent in aged individuals (Hildemann and Walford, 1966; Teague et al., 1970; Naor et al., 1976; Meredith et al., 1979). The frequency of cancer also increases with advancing age, suggesting a cause-effect relationship with the decline of immune potential (Walford, 1969).

(1)

Does all this mean that the immune system plays a role in the aging process? The age-related decline in efficiency is not unique to the immune system; it has been found to occur for most other bodily systems. The immune system, however, is entrusted with the preservation of the integrity of organs and tissues. It is possible, therefore, that its deterioration may lead to secondary lesions in other organ systems which, together, constitute what we call "aging". This is, in essence, the claim made by the Immunologic Theory of Aging that was advanced several years ago by Roy Walford (Walford, 1969). I hold no brief for this theory. It may or may not be sound. Certain observations are at least consistent with the theory. For example, many of the so-called "diseases of aging," such as senile amyloidosis, late-occurring cancers, renal disease, diabetes, and others involve a compromised immune response. Moreover, epidemiological studies have suggested that, in the elderly, decreased immune competence and the presence of autoantibodies identify subpopulations at high risk of early death (MacKay, 1972; Roberts-Thomson et al., 1974). Whether we view the Immunologic Theory of Aging with favor or disfavor, it is incumbent upon us who are working in experimental immunogerontology to attempt to test the theory. If we don't do it, nobody will.

(2)

This brings me to my second question: What is the role of the experimental immunogerontologist?

I have already given one answer to this question. We must attempt to test experimentally the hypothesis that the immune system plays a primary role in the aging process. To put it in other words, is the immune system a biological clock?

On a less theoretical, but equally fundamental level, we should try to take immunogerontology beyond the phenomenological phase and explore the mechanisms that lead to the decline in the immune potential of aged individuals. The immune system is complex and is subject to complex cellular and chemical regulatory factors. Fortunately, immunology, especially the immunology of the mouse, has made great strides forward and we now begin to understand the complexity of the immune system and to be able to assay for the integrity of many immunologic functions. Does aging affect certain functions more than others, certain regulatory processes more than others? The answers to these questions are within reach. Powerful analytical tools, such as the radioimmunoassay, reagents, such as hybridoma-derived monoclonal antibodies, and made-to-order experimental animals, such as mutant and congenic mouse strains, are available to the immunogerontologist in his attempts to answer these questions. The other ingredient, the ingenuity of the experimentalist, has long been available.

As stated earlier, a compromised or malfunctioning immune system has been associated with many of the diseases of aging. The relationship between these diseases and the immune system is an important area of immunogerontological investigation. Again, the mouse model has proven useful and will continue to do so. For example, studies on autoimmunity have benefitted from the availability of autoimmunity-prone mouse strains such as the NZB, the NZB/W, and the newly developed MRL and BXSB.

How should the immunogerontologist proceed in fulfilling his role? Obviously, there is no single answer to this question. In fact, any attempt to chart a course of action too precisely is likely to restrict and hinder the creativity which is the hallmark of the imaginative research scientist. I will, however, list certain areas of research which I consider particularly important or relevant.

First, I would like to say a word on the choice of the experimental animals. Mice and rats have been used extensively in immunogerontology for obvious reasons. The similarity of the mouse immune system to that of man, the availability of inbred strains of mice, the susceptibility to diseases of aging, the short lifespan, are all features that make the mouse the animal of choice for gerontological studies. It must be emphasized that immunogerontological investigations must include truly senescent animals, that is, animals from relatively disease-free, long-lived strains which have at least reached the age corresponding to the median lifespan of the strain (Walford, 1976). Conclusions based only on extrapolations of earlier events may well be invalid. This is not to say that short-lived strains should not be used for particular investigations. But it must be kept in mind that animals such as, for example, the NZB mice, have ongoing pathological processes and may or may not represent valid models for similar pathological processes that occur in senescence.

One set of experiments that seems to me to be particularly relevant is the dissection and analysis of the age-related behavior of the components of the immune system. Does the functional decline of the various components of the immune system proceed at the same rate? Or is there one or more components which deteriorate faster than the others? Just as the immune system may be a biological clock, a particular component of the immune system may be an immunological clock. The thymus appears to be a good candidate for a rate-limiting organ. Perhaps we are only as old as our thymus. But the thymic functions are themselves complex, as they include the generation and differentiation of an ever-increasing number of cell subpopulations as well as the secretion of hormones. We should make an effort to learn how these various elements change with advancing age, especially since the most prominent feature of the senescent immune system appears to be its deregulation (autoimmunity, immune dysfunctions, etc.), and the thymus and its products are heavily involved in immunoregulation.

The relation between nutrition, immunity, and lifespan is another area that deserves intensive investigation. Startling results have already been acquired by prolonged nutritional caloric restriction. Lifespan has been lengthened in both normal (Gerbase-DeLima et al., 1975) and autoimmune (Fernandes et al., 1978) mice, whose immune systems have remained youthful in spite of the chronological age of the host. Was a well preserved immune system the cause of longevity in these animals? Or was the immune system well preserved because the mice lived so long? These are fascinating questions, but difficult to answer.

The immune system does not exist in a vacuum. It interacts with, and is regulated by, other systems, especially the neuroendocrine system. One needs only mention the intense research activity that has centered on the thymic hormones and their activity on T cell differentiation. In general, the level of thymic hormone decreases with advancing age. Whether this observation affords an opportunity for corrective measures intended to restore function to an aging immune system by administration of thymic hormones, remains to be seen. The elegant experiments of Fabris (Farbis, 1977) with the pituitary dwarf mice have demonstrated the profound influence of the hypophysis on the immune system. Recent work has shown that neuroendocrine influences modulate the immune function (Strom et al., 1981). The prevalence of systemic lupus erythematosus among females, in both humans and mice, hints at a role for sex hormones in this autoimmune condition. In fact, it has been found that androgens suppress and estrogens accelerate the disease (Talal et al., 1981). I have chosen these few examples to emphasize that the study of the interactions between the endocrine and the immune systems should be an important and potentially fruitful area of research for the immunogerontologist.

That lifespan is under genetic control is both self-evident and accepted. Only recently, however, has this notion acquired more precise meaning. Studies by Walford (Walford, 1980) have uncovered a correlation between the major histocompatibility complex haplotype and maximum lifespan in mice. The mechanisms by which the MHC influences lifespan are largely unknown, and may or may not involve the immune system. However, since the control of the immune responses is one of the major functions of this genetic system, the possible relevance of these studies to immunogerontology should not be neglected.

It would not be terribly useful to continue this list of areas of investigation of potential interest to immunogerontology. Prophecy is a risky business, and I am certainly not in a position to guess where the future advances in immunogerontology will come from. The only thing that I am reasonably sure of is that there will be advances in our understanding of the process of aging, and that immunology will play a role in the progress that will be made.

At this point, then, I would like to ask the last of my questions: What are the ultimate goals of experimental immunogerontology? As I see it, there are two major goals. The first is to put the hypothesis that the deterioration of the immune system is a primary cause of aging to experimental test. The second is to find means to delay the age-related decline of immune potential.

How to approach these problems is, of course, a question that the investigator will have to resolve for himself. Indeed, success will depend in large measure on the ability and ingenuity of the scientists who are presently working in this field and of those now working in other areas whom we may be able to attract to immunogerontology if we argue convincingly that this is an important and potentially rewarding science. I suggest, however, that a demonstration of the primary role of the immune system in aging will require the experimental prolongation of lifespan by immunologic interventions shown to maintain the integrity of the immune system over time. If we can accomplish this, we will also have fulfilled the second of the goals I have mentioned earlier.

What are the prospects of success? I believe that there is reasonable hope that we may be able to delay the age-related decline of the immune function and perhaps even to effect a measure of rejuvenation of the immune system. My optimism stems from the finding that certain components of the immune system age faster than others. For example, my collaborators and I have found that an exaggerated suppressor function appears in relatively young mice whose B cell and T helper cell functions are still moderately good (Segre and Segre, 1977; Segre et al., 1981). We are now planning to attempt to depress the suppressor function by administration of anti-I-J serum. Whether this will have an effect on the immune potential of the mice, or even on their longevity remains to be seen.

Acknowledgment: The author's work cited was supported by grant No. AG 00451 from the National Institutes on Aging.

REFERENCES:

DeKruyff, R.H., Rinnooy Kan, E.A., Weksler, M.E. and Siskind, G.W., 1980. Effect of aging on T-cell tolerance induction. Cell. Immunol., 56: 58-67.

Fabris, N., 1977. Hormones and aging. In: T. Makinodan and E. Yunis (Editors), Immunology and Aging. Plenum, New York, pp. 73-89.

Fernandes, G., Yunis, E.J., Miranda, M., Smith, J. and Good, R.A., 1978. Nutritional inhibition of genetically determined renal disease and autoimmunity with prolongation of life in kdkd mice. Proc. Natl. Acad. Sci. USA, 75: 2888-2892.

Gerbase-DeLima, M., Liu, R.K., Cheney, K.E., Mickey, R. and Walford, R.L., 1975. Immune function and survival in a long-lived mouse strain subjected to undernutrition. Gerontologia, 21: 184-202.

Hildemann, W.H. and Walford, R.L., 1966. Autoimmunity in relation to aging as measured by agar plaque technique. Proc. Soc. Exp. Biol. Med., 123: 417-421.

Kiessling, R. and Haller, O., 1978. Natural killer cells in the mouse: An alternative immune surveillance mechanism? Contemp. Topics Immunobiol., 8: 171-201.

MacKay, I.R., 1972. Aging and immunological function in man. Gerontologia, 18: 239-245.

Makinodan, T. and Kay, M.M.B., 1980. Age influence on the immune system. Adv. Immunol., 29:287-330.

McIntosh, K.R. and Segre, D., 1976. B- and T-cell tolerance induction in young-adult and old mice. Cell. Immunol. 27:230-239.

Meredith, P., Kristie, J. and Walford, R.L., 1979. Aging increases expression of LPS-induced autoantibody-secreting B cells. J. Immunol., 123:87-91.

Naor, D., Bonavida, B. and Walford, R.L., 1976. Autoimmunity and aging: The age-related response of a long-lived strain to trinitrophenylated syngeneic mouse red blood cells. J. Immunol., 117: 2204-2208.

Roberts-Thomson, E.C., Wittingham, S., Youngchayud, U. and MacKay, I.R., 1974. Aging, immune response, and mortality. Lancet, 2: 368-370.

Segre, D. and Segre, M. 1977. Age-related changes in B and T lymphocytes and decline of the humoral immune responsiveness in aged mice. Mech. Age. Develop., 6: 115-129.

Segre, D., Liu, J.J. and Segre, D., 1981. T-helper, T-suppressor and B-cell functions in aged mice. This volume.

Strom, T.B., Smith, K.A., Lane, M.A. and Helderman, J.H., 1981. Does age-associated deterioration in T cell regulation by neuroendocrine agonists and T cell growth factor cause immunosenescence? In: D. Segre and L. Smith (Editors), Immunological Aspects of Aging. Marcel Dekker, New York, in press.

Talal, N., Dauphinee, M. and Roubinian, J.R., 1981. The effect of sex hormones and thymosin on autoimmunity. In: D. Segre and L. Smith (Editors), Immunological Aspects of Aging. Marcel Dekker, New York, in press.

Teague, P., Yunis, E., Fish, A., Stutman, O. and Good, R., 1970. Auto-immune phenomena and renal disease in mice. Role of thymectomy, aging, and involution of thymic capacity. Lab. Invest., 22: 121-130.

Walford, R.L., 1969. The Immunologic Theory of Aging. Munksgaard, Copenhagen.

Walford, R.L., 1976. When is a mouse old? J. Immunol., 117: 352-353.

Walford, R.L., 1980. Immunology and aging. Am. J. Clin. Path., 74: 247-253.

T-HELPER, T-SUPPRESSOR AND B-CELL FUNCTIONS IN AGING MICE

Mariangela Segre, Jiuan J. Liu and Diego Segre
Department of Veterinary Pathobiology
University of Illinois
Urbana, Illinois, USA

ABSTRACT

We have analyzed the lymphocyte function in mice from 4 to 30 months of age. T-suppressor function was assessed from the ability of test spleen cells to suppress the secondary PFC response of spleen cells from young mice. T-helper function was assayed as the capacity of test cells to become activated following stimulation with carrier-anticarrier immune complexes. B-cell function was measured from the PFC response of test cells to the T-independent antigen DNP-Ficoll. While B-cell and T-helper cell functions declined at a constant rate from 4 to 30 months of age, suppressor function increased at 15 months of age and remained elevated thereafter.

INTRODUCTION

It has long been known that the activity of the immune system declines in an age-related fashion after reaching a peak in young-adult animals (for a recent review see Makinodan and Kay, 1980). This pattern applies to both the humoral and the cell-mediated immune responses. Even though much of the early work was of a descriptive, phenomenological nature, important insights into the mechanisms of the age-related immuno-logical deficit were gained, particularly through the work of Makinodan and collaborators (reviewed in Makinodan et al., 1971). With the reali-zation of the complexities of cell interactions in the immune response and the comparatively recent availability of techniques that allow the selective separation and removal of immunologically relevant cell types, it has become possible to undertake the cellular analysis of the humoral immunologic deficiency of senescence. Earlier work from this laboratory (Segre and Segre, 1977) presented data suggesting that an increase in T-suppressor function is the first immunologic lesion of aging mice, and that this is followed by a decrease in T-helper function and finally by a loss of B-cell function. These conclusions were only tentative, because the sequence in which the lymphocyte dysfunctions occur was inferred from the frequency of each dysfunction in senescent mice. In addition, T-helper function was assayed without removing T-suppressor cells from the lymphocyte population.

In this report we describe the functional behavior of T-helper, T-suppressor and B-cells from young, middle-aged and senescent mice. T-helper function was assessed under conditions which prevent the generation of T-suppressor cells (Ding et al., 1979).

MATERIALS AND METHODS

Female BC3Fl hybrid mice (median lifespan approximately 30 months) were used as spleen cell donors. Swiss Webster female retired breeders of the ICR strain were used as recipients of Millipore diffusion chambers. Keyhole limpet hemocyanin (KLH) and human gamma globulin (HGG) were dinitrophenylated as described by Little and Eisen (1967). DNP-Ficoll was purchased from Biosearch, San Rafael, California. The methods for propagation of spleen cells in diffusion chambers (Segre and Segre, 1972) and for the detection and enumeration of DNP-specific plaque forming cells (PFC) (Miller and Segre, 1972; Segre and Segre, 1976a) that have been previously described were followed in this work, with the exception that the recipient ICR mice were given 8 mg cyclophosphamide intraperitoneally 24 hours before implantation of the diffusion chambers, instead of X-irradiation.

Single cell suspensions were prepared from spleens of individual BC3Fl mice of approximately 4, 15, 22 and 30 months of age. The T-suppressor, T-helper and B-cell functions of each spleen suspension were measured as follows.

T-suppressor function. A single cell suspension was prepared from spleens of young (4 to 6 months of age) BC3Fl mice that had been primed 3 to 5 weeks earlier by intraperitoneal injection of 100 µg DNP-HGG adsorbed on bentonite (Rittenberg and Pratt, 1969). Fifty nanograms of soluble DNP-HGG were added per each 15×10^6 viable primed cells. Fifteen million cells were then introduced into each of 2 to 4 diffusion chambers. Two to four additional diffusion chambers were filled with 15×10^6 primed, antigen-stimulated cells to which an equal number of viable cells to be assayed for suppressor activity had been added. The chambers were implanted into the peritoneal cavity of cyclophosphamide-treated ICR recipient mice. After 6 to 7 days the cells were recovered from the chambers and assayed for DNP-specific indirect PFC. Suppressor activity of the test cells was manifested by a reduction in the number of PFC found in the chambers containing primed cells and test cells by comparison to the number of PFC in chambers containing primed cells only. Although the T-cell nature of the suppressor cells was not determined in this investigation, previous work (Segre and Segre, 1976b) had shown that, under similar conditions, suppression was abrogated by treatment of the cells with anti-Thy-1 serum and complement.

T-helper function. A portion of each individual spleen cell suspension from the test mice was passed through a column of nylon wool (Julius et al., 1973). Ten million nylon wool non-adherent viable cells were stimulated with immune complexes consisting of 50 ng KLH premixed with 0.1 ml of a rabbit anti-KLH serum diluted 1:100, as described by Ding et al. (1979). The cells were then cultured in diffusion chambers for 6 days. Spleen cells from young BC3Fl mice that had been primed with 100 µg DNP-HGG adsorbed on bentonite 3 to 5 weeks earlier were treated with monoclonal anti-Thy-1.2 antibody (New England Nuclear, Boston, Massachusetts) and complement. Fifteen million viable, DNP-HGG-primed, T-cell-depleted spleen cells were supplemented or not with 1.5×10^6 test cells recovered from the chambers, boosted with 50 ng DNP-KLH and cultured in each of 2 to 4 diffusion chambers. Seven to eight days later the cultures were assayed for DNP-specific indirect PFC. A significant increase in the number of PFC obtained in the cultures supplemented with the test cells over the number of PFC in unsupplemented cultures indicated that the test cells contained activated, carrier-specific T-helper cells. The ratio of the mean number of PFC in supplemented cultures to the mean number of PFC in unsupplemented cultures was taken as a measure of the extent of T-helper cell activation by immune complexes (Ding et al., 1979).

B-cell function. Nylon wool adherent cells were recovered from the nylon wool used to prepare the cells to be tested for T-helper cell function (see above). The nylon wool was removed from the column and soaked in a petri dish containing tissue culture medium 199. The nylon wool was gently teased apart with forceps and shaken on a reciprocating shaker for 5 minutes at room temperature. Fifteen million viable cells were cultured in a diffusion chamber with 50 ng DNP-Ficoll for 7 or 8 days. The cells were recovered and assayed for DNP-specific direct PFC. The mean number of PFC obtained from 2 to 4 replicate cultures was taken as a measure of B-cell function of the test cells.

RESULTS

The plot of percent suppression vs age of the donor mice (Fig. 1, bottom panel) showed that suppressor activity increased rapidly from 4 months to 15 months of age. Thereafter, suppressor activity increased only slightly. The difference in suppressor activity between the test cells from 4 months old mice and those from each of the other age groups was highly statistically significant, whereas there were no significant differences among the suppressor activities of test cells from the 15, 22 and 30 months age group.

The T-helper activity of the test cells (Fig. 1, middle panel) decreased at a constant rate from 4 to 30 months of age. There was a highly significant negative correlation between the age of the donor mice and their T-helper activity ($r = 0.99$).

The B-cell activity of the test cells (Fig. 1, top panel) also decreased at a constant rate from the youngest to the oldest age group. In this case also, a highly significant negative correlation was found between the age of the donor mice and their B-cell activity ($r = 0.99$).

Some of the mice from the oldest age group (30 months) had grossly enlarged spleens. The mean number of nucleated cells/spleen in these mice was 12.77×10^8 vs 2.54×10^8 nucleated cells/spleen for mice of the same age with normal size spleen. Spleen cells from the mice with splenomegaly had no detectable T-suppressor, T-helper and B-cell function (Fig. 1).

DISCUSSION

The results reported here confirm the age-related increase in suppressor activity that had been found in this (Segre and Segre, 1976b) and other laboratories (Makinodan et al., 1976; Goidl et al., 1976; Callard and Basten, 1978; DeKruyff et al., 1980). In particular, our results indicate that the increase in suppressor activity occurs at a relatively early age, a finding also reported by DeKruyff et al. (1980). This finding is in agreement with our earlier suggestion, based on the frequency of the immune defects found in senescent mice, that the increase in suppression function is the earliest age-related immunologic change (Segre and Segre, 1977).

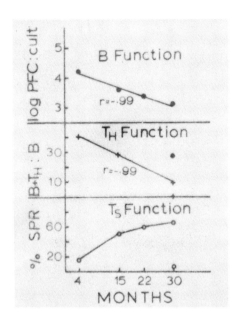

Figure 1. Age-related changes in lymphocyte functions. The percent suppression (% SPR, bottom panel), T-helper cell activation (the ratio of the PFC response of mixed cultures of T and B cells to that of B cells only [B+T_H:B] middle panel) and the B-cell response per culture (log PFC:cult, top panel) are plotted against the age, in months, of the cell donors. In each panel, the points that fall outside the connecting lines indicate the response of cells from 30 months old donor mice with enlarged spleens.

T-helper and B-cell functions were also found to decline with age, but the decline occurred at a constant rate throughout the life of the mice. Although deficiencies in T-helper cells in senescent mice have been inferred (Segre and Segre, 1977; Makinodan et al., 1976; Krosgrud and Perkins, 1977; Weksler et al., 1978), the investigations of this parameter and the interpretation of the results have been complicated by the likely presence of suppressor cells in the cell population being tested. In the work described here, we have taken advantage of our own finding that immune complexes made at the appropriate antigen:antibody ratio activate carrier-specific T-helper cells, but do not generate suppressor cells (Ding et al., 1979). The results clearly show an age-related decline in the T-helper function. They do not establish whether the decline was due to reduced numbers of resting T cells, to a lack of responsiveness of these cells to immunologic stimuli, or to a decrease in the number of effector cells generated by each resting T cell. Further work will be necessary to distinguish among these and other possibilities.

We have reported earlier (Segre and Segre, 1977) that the B-cell function of senescent mice was often vigorous. In this work, however, we found that the B-cell function declines at a constant rate with advancing age. The discrepancy between these two findings is probably related to the assay used to measure B-cell function. In our earlier work (Segre and Segre, 1977), we measured the response to a T-dependent antigen of T-cell depleted cultures that were supplemented with carrier specific T-helper cells from young mice. In this work, we measured the response of B-cells to a T-independent antigen. The present results are in agreement with those of Callard et al. (1977) and of DeKruyff et al. (1980) who found an age-related decline in the responsiveness to the T-independent antigens pneumococcal polysaccharide type III and DNP conjugated to polyacrylamide beads, respectively. In contrast, Naor et al. (1976) found that the magnitude of the PFC response to the T-independent antigen TNP-syngeneic RBC was not reduced by aging. However, they suggested that this was due to an age-related immunoloregulatory defect which allowed the B-cells to respond to a modified self-component, similarly to what is assumed to occur for the increased frequency of autoantibodies in senescent mice.

The finding that spleen cells from old mice with severely enlarged spleens lacked detectable immunologic activity was unexpected. Jaroslow et al. (1975) reported that cells from the enlarged spleen of aged BC3Fl mice with reticulum cell sarcoma and generalized lymphoma suppressed the in vitro response of normal spleen cells to SRBC. Cells from a transplantable lymphoma were also immunosuppressive. However, no suppressor activity was detected in the spleen cells from old mice with splenomegaly in the present study. The other immunologic functions that were measured were also lacking. The mice were not visibly unhealthy. Possibly, their immunologic needs were satisfied by lymphoid organs other than the spleen.

Finally, the finding that the increase in T-suppressor function occurs at an age when the T-helper and the B-cell functions are still relatively vigorous suggests that immunologic interventions designed to specifically inhibit T-suppressor cells may be a valid approach to rejuvenation of the immune system.

Acknowledgment. This work was supported by grant No. AG 00451 from the National Institute on Aging.

REFERENCES

Callard, R.E, Basten, A. and Waters, L.K., 1977. Immune function in aged mice. II. B cell function. Cell. Immunol., 31: 26–36.
Callard, R.E. and Basten, A., 1978. Immune function in aged mice. IV. Loss of T cell and B cell function in thymus-dependent antibody responses. Eur. J. Immunol., 8: 552–558.
DeKruyff, R.H., Kim, Y.T., Siskind, G.W. and Weksler, M.E., 1980. Age-related changes in the in vitro immune response: Increased suppressor activity in immature and aged mice. J. Immunol., 125: 142–147.
Ding, D.-H., Segre, M. and Segre, D., 1979. Activation of helper T Cells by immune complexes. Cell. Immunol., 46: 281–296.
Goidl, E.A., Innes, J.B. and Weksler, M.E., 1976. Immunological studies of Aging. II. Loss of IgG and high avidity plaque-forming cells and increased suppressor activity in aging mice. J. Exp. Med., 144: 1037–1048.
Jaroslow, B.N., Suhrbier, K.M., Fry, R.J.M. and Taylor, S.A., 1975. In vitro suppression of immunocompetent cells by lymphomas from aging mice. J. Nat. Cancer Inst., 54: 1427–1431.
Julius, M.H., Simpson, F. and Herzenberg, L.A., 1973. A rapid method for the isolation of functional thymus-derived murine lymphocytes. Eur. J. Immunol., 3: 645–649.
Krosgrud, R.L. and Perkins, E.H., 1977. Age-related changes in T-cell function. J. Immunol., 118: 1607–1611.
Little, J.R. and Eisen, H.N., 1967. Preparation of immunogenic 2,4-dinitrophenyl and 2,4,6-trinitrophenyl proteins. In: C.A. Williams and M.W. Chase (editors), Methods in Immunology and Immunochemistry. Vol. I. Academic Press, New York, pp. 128–133.
Makinodan, T., Perkins, E.H. and Chen, M.G., 1971. Immunologic activity of the aged. Adv. Gerontol. Res., 3: 171–198.
Makinodan, T., Albright, J.W., Good, P.I., Peter, C.P. and Heidrick, M.L., 1976. Reduced humoral immune activity in long-lived mice: An approach to elucidating its mechanisms. Immunology 31: 903–911.
Makinodan, T. and Kay, M.B., 1980. Age influence on the immune system. Adv. Immunol., 29: 287–330.
Miller, G.W. and Segre, D., 1972. Determination of relative affinity and heterogeneity of mouse Anti-DNP antibodies by a plaque inhibition technique. J. Immunol., 109: 74–83.

Naor, D., Bonavida, B. and Walford, R.L., 1976. Autoimmunity and aging: The age-related response of a long-lived strain to trinitrophenylated syngeneic mouse red blood cells. J. Immunol., 117: 2204-2208.

Rittenberg, M.B. and Pratt, K.L., 1969. Anti-trinitrophenyl (TNP) plaque assay. Primary response of Balb/c mice to soluble and particulate immunogens. Proc. Soc. Exp. Biol. Med., 132: 575-581.

Segre, M. and Segre, D., 1972. Anti-DNP hemolytic plaques by mouse spleen cells in diffusion chambers. Immunol. Commun., 1: 143-153.

Segre, D. and Segre, M., 1976a. Visualization of plaque forming cells in agar plates stained with O-tolidine. J. Immunol. Meth., 12: 197-198.

Segre, D. and Segre, M., 1976b. Humoral immunity in aged mice. II. Increased suppressor T cell activity in immunologically deficient old mice. J. Immunol., 116: 735-738.

Segre, D. and Segre, M., 1977. Age-related changes in B and T lymphocytes and decline of the humoral immune responsiveness in aged mice. Mech. Age. Develop., 6: 115-129.

Weksler, M.E., Innes, J.B. and Goldstein, G., 1978. Immunological studies of aging. IV. The contribution of thymic involution to the immune deficiencies of aging mice and reversal with thymopoietin. J. Exp. Med., 148: 996-1006.

86

MOUSE T AND B LYMPHOCYTE SUBPOPULATIONS:
CHANGES WITH AGE

J.J. Haaijman, J.M. Ure and H.S. Micklem

Institute for Experimental Gerontology TNO, Rijswijk (ZH)

The Netherlands and Department of Zoology

University of Edinburgh, Edinburgh, U.K.

SUMMARY.

Monoclonal antibodies to murine Thy-1, Lyt-1, Lyt-2, ThB, IgM and IgD antigenic determinants were used in conjunction with the fluorescence activated cell sorter and fluorescence microscopy to analyse T and B cell subpopulations in early postnatal and adult life. T cell subpopulations were also analysed in aged (up to 30 month old) animals. The frequency of $Lyt\text{-}2^+$ cells, in relation to total T lymphocytes as defined by the possession of surface Thy-1 antigen, was similar in 10-day-old and adult spleen (30-40%). Thus there was no evidence for a predominantly $Lyt\text{-}1^+, 2^+$ population early in life.

Old mice showed considerable variability, but the following trends were noted: a decrease in the frequency of $Thy\text{-}1^+$ cells in thymus and peripheral lymphoid tissue, with a concomitant increase in B cells carrying surface immunoglobulin (sIg) determinants; and an increase in the Lyt-2/Thy-1 ratio in lymph nodes, peripheral blood and (less markedly) spleen. This was interpreted in terms of a decline in homeostatic control of T cell subsets with, frequently, a selective loss of $Lyt\text{-}1^+, 2^-$ cells. It may be associated with the relatively high T-suppressor activity reported in some old mice. B lymphocyte ontogeny as analysed by two-colour fluorescence of surface Ig determinants in the FACS, showed a progression from almost exclusively IgM^{++}/IgD^- cells in 10-day-old spleen to the IgM^+/IgD^+ population of adults, with IgM^{++}/IgD^+ cells as a possible intermediate stage.

INTRODUCTION

Subpopulations of T and B lymphocytes can be delineated on the basis both of their functions and of their possession of various antigenic macromolecules in their cell membranes. Thus, various functional T cell subsets have been operationally identified and separated with the aid of cytotoxic antibodies to the antigens Lyt-1, Lyt-2 and Lyt-3 (Cantor & Boyse, 1975 a,b; Feldmann et al., 1975; Shiku et al., 1975).

Similarly the functional capacities of B cells have been associated with the presence of particular classes of immunoglobulin (Ig) on their surface (Abney et al., 1978).

More recently, antibodies have been used not only as cytotoxic depleting agents, but also as tools for the enrichment of antigen-carrying cells by such techniques as fluorescence-activated cell sorting (Herzenberg and Herzenberg, 1978) and panning (Wysocki & Sato, 1978).

The advent of monoclonal antibodies, with their virtues of known specificity and consistency, has given new impetus to studies of this kind. In conjunction with the fluorescence activated cell sorter (FACS) they also provide important analytical tools for the demonstration and relative quantification of the respective antigens on cell surfaces. In this paper we summarize the changes observed by FACS analysis and fluorescence microscopy in the subset composition of murine T and B lymphocyte subpopulations during post-natal ontogeny and during senescence.

MATERIALS AND METHODS

Mice

BALB/cNHz, SJL/JHz and (BALB/c × SJL/J)F1 mice were bred and maintained at the Genetics Department, Stanford University, School of Medicine, and CBA/ca mice at the Zoology Department, University of Edinburgh. Females only were used. All mice received a pelleted diet and tap-water ad libitum.

Antibodies

The preparation and characterization of monoclonal rat antibodies directed against murine Thy-1, Lyt-1, Lyt-2, Lyt-3 and ThB antigens have been described previously (Ledbetter & Herzenberg, 1979; Ledbetter et al., 1980).

In addition, monoclonal antibodies to murine IgD (Oi et al., 1978) and IgM (Haaijman, 1981) were used. These reagents were either directly labelled with a fluorochrome (FITC: fluorescein isothiocyanate or TRITC: tetramethyl rhodamine isothiocyanate) or used with a FITC conjugated second-step reagent (a predominantly IgG1 fraction of hyperimmune SJL/J mouse anti-rat/Ig serum), or conjugated with biotin, TRITC-conjugated avidin (Bayer & Wilchek, 1974) being used as the second-step reagent. A FITC-conjugated goat anti-mouse/Ig (Nordic Immunological Laboratories, Tilburg, The Netherlands), was used to enumerate surface Ig (sIg)-bearing cells.

Cell suspensions

Spleen, thymus and lymph node suspensions were prepared by gentle dissociation in RPMI 1640 medium containing 2-5% heat-inactivated foetal calf serum (FCS), 0.1% NaN3 and (in some experiments) 20mM HEPES. In preparations for fluorescence microscopy erythrocytes were removed by lysis in glycerol. Peripheral blood lymphocytes were prepared by centrifugation on Lympholyte-M (Cedar Lane Laboratories, Hornby, Ontario, Canada). Cells were washed twice by centrifugation and their number and percentage viability were determined by staining an aliquot with acridine orange and ethidium bromide (1 microgram/ml of each) and counting with a fluorescence microscope. The cells were kept at approximately 4°C throughout the preparation and staining procedures.

Staining

One million viable cells in 25-50 μl of medium were incubated for 30 minutes on melting ice in 96-well flexible Microtiter plates with monoclonal antibodies, either unlabelled or fluorochrome-conjugated. For indirect staining, the cells were washed two to three times with 150 μl medium. Then, 2 μl FITC-conjugated SJL mouse anti-rat/Ig was added in a total volume of 50 μl and the cells were incubated for a further 30 minutes on ice. For two-colour staining of sIg, cells were incubated first with a mixture of anti-IgM and biotin-conjugated anti-IgD and then with a mixture of FITC-mouse anti-rat/Ig and TRITC-avidin.

Finally, the stained cells were washed twice and either examined directly in a fluorescence microscope or diluted to a volume of about 1 ml for FACS analysis.

FACS Analysis

Scatter and fluorescence profiles of each sample were obtained with a modified fluorescence activated cell sorter (FACS-2: Becton-Dickinson FACS Systems, Sunnyvale, California) using logarithmic amplification of the fluorescence signals (Herzenberg & Herzenberg, 1978). Low-angle light scatter gates were used to exclude the fluorescence signals from objects falling outside the scatter range characteristic of viable cells. The percentage of cells falling within a given fluorescence range was determined by integration from profiles based on 10,000 cells.

RESULTS

1.   Ontogeny of T lymphocytes

   a) Spleen

   Data on the percentage of BALB/c cells stained by monoclonal antibodies to Thy-1, Lyt-1 and Lyt-2 are shown in Table 1. At ten days
after birth very few T cells were present in the spleen. The proportion
rose rapidly between three and five weeks of age, when the adult level
was attained. There was an apparent tendency for the ratio of Lyt-2$^+$ to
Thy-1$^+$ cells to rise with increasing age, but the increase was not drama-
tic and was not observed in another mouse strain (Haaijman et al., 1981).

TABLE 1 - THE DEVELOPMENT OF LYMPHOCYTE SUBPOPULATIONS IN BALB/c SPLEEN
Percentage of positive cells

Age (days)	Thy-1	Lyt-1	Lyt-2
10	3	5	1
20	6	10	2
35	22	26	8
60	26	29	10
140	28	34	12

   A previous report that most splenic T cells in nursling mice carry
Lyt-2 (Cantor and Boyse, 1975a) was not confirmed. Moreover, the frequency of T cells before the twentieth day of life was much lower than
reported by Cantor and Boyse. The frequency of Lyt-1$^+$ cells was consistently rather higher than that of Thy-1$^+$; this agrees with a previous
report that all Thy-1$^+$ cells carried some Lyt-1 and that, in addition, a
few Thy-1$^-$, Lyt-1$^+$ were detectable (Ledbetter et al., 1980). The nature
of these latter cells, which are found in what are generally regarded as
'B' areas in the spleen, has yet to be elucidated. Preliminary data indicate that Thy-1$^+$, Lyt-1$^+$ cells are much more frequent in the lymph nodes
than in the spleen within the first week after birth, but the relative
frequency of Lyt-2$^+$ cells has yet to be established.

b) Thymus

Four hours after birth the thymus contained a population of cells which was almost homogenous with respect to the frequency and density of expression of Thy-1, Lyt-1 and Lyt-2 antigens. The great majority of cells resembled those which are present in the cortex of the adult thymus and which are cortisone-sensitive, in being Thy-1$^+$, Lyt-1$^+$, Lyt-2$^+$ and carrying a high concentration of Thy-1 and relatively little Lyt-1 on their surface (Ledbetter et al., 1980; Potter et al., 1980). By 24 hours clear evidence of a second population, resembling the medullary cortisone-resistant population of the adult was visible. As shown in Table 2 this population, characterized by relatively low Thy-1 and high Lyt-1 densities increased progressively, reaching an adult frequency by four days. It is noteworthy that during this developmental period the frequency of high Lyt-1 cells was consistently greater than that of low Thy-1 cells; indeed, up to 42% of thymic cells in young adults were classified as high Lyt-1 on the basis fo FACS analysis. Since the cortisone resistant medullary population comprised only about 10% of thymocytes, it follows that some 30% of cortical thymocytes must belong in the high Lyt-1 class. The density of Lyt-2 per cells differed only over a narrow range and no age-related shift was discerned.

TABLE 2 - THE DIFFERENTIATION OF THYMOCYTE SUBPOPULATIONS IN BALB/c MICE

Age	Percentage of cells with	
	low Thy-1	high Lyt-1
4 hr	3	14
24 hr	14	32
4 day	21	38
7 day	17	n.d.
60 day	19	42

The pattern of development of Thy-1 and Lyt-1 expression is most easily explicable on the basis that low Thy-1, high Lyt-1 cells are derived from high Thy-1, low Lyt-1. However, proof is lacking, and the view that medullary thymocytes are derived from cortical precursors has been disputed by some authors (Weissman et al., 1975; Stutman, 1977).

The expression of the ThB antigen was somewhat surprising. In the adult, ThB is expressed on cortical thymocytes and B cells, but not on spleen colony-forming cells, medullary thymocytes or T cells (Eckhardt & Herzenberg, 1980; Haaijman et al., 1981). This distribution gave rise to the speculation that ThB might be present on a common bone marrow progenitor for B and T lymphocyte lineages. However, expression of ThB on thymocytes achieved the adult frequency only slowly.

THYMUS : ThB STAINING

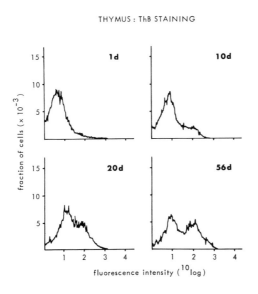

Figure 1. The expression of ThB by developing BALB/c thymocytes. Histograms were obtained with a fluorescence activated cell sorter equiped with a logarithmic amplifier. Gates were set to exclude any dead cells.

Less than 10% of BALB/c thymocytes carried the antigen at 24 hours of age and only 16% on day 7. The adult frequency (about 50%) was reached before the eight week of life, but the time was not precisely determined.

Although this probably argues against ThB as a differentiation marker for lymphocyte progenitors, since the antigen might then be expected on most neonatal thymocytes, it does not rule out the idea: cortical thymocytes might lose the antigen more rapidly during neonatal than during adult T cell differentiation. More work is needed on the significance of ThB as a differentiation antigen.

2. Ontogeny of B lymphocytes

The kinetics of appearance of IgM and IgD, the two main immuno-globulin isotypes of lymphocyte surfaces, are still poorly understood although IgD appears later in development that IgM (Vitetta et al., 1975). Using a monoclonal rat anti-mouse/IgM (Haaijman, 1981) and mouse allotypic anti-IgD (Oi et al., 1978) antibodies we found, as Goding et al. (1977) has done, that the first surface IgM-carrying cells stained brightly for IgM and very dully, if at all, for IgD (designated $M^{++}D^-$ cells).

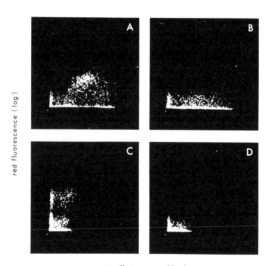

Figure 2. Two-colour analysis of sIgM and sIgD on 28-day-old BALB/c spleen.
Spleen cells were incubated as explained in the text. The green fluorescence signifies sIgM density, red fluorescence that of sIgD. Each single dot in the figure represents an individual cell. The FACS was set to analyse only lymphocyte-sized cells. a) cells stained for sIgM and sIgD; b) control: cells stained for sIgM only; c) control: cells stained for sIgD only; d) control: unstained cells.

Three to six weeks after birth, cells gradually appeared which stained relatively dully for IgM and were positive for IgD (designated M^+D^+). Two-colour FACS analysis of four week old BALB/c spleen using indirect stains (rat anti-mouse/IgM followed by FITC-conjugated mouse anti-rat/IgG, and biotin-conjugated anti-IgD followed by TRITC-conjugated avidin) distinguished three discrete populations of surface Ig-carrying cells: $M^{++}D^-$, $M^{++}D^+$ and M^+D^+. In adult spleen the great majority of B cells belong to the third category. A logical development sequence would be $M^{++}D^- \rightarrow M^{++}D^+ \rightarrow M^+D^+$. A complicating element in this picture is that there is some heterogeneity of staining intensity within the M^+D^+ category, M and D being positively correlated. It remains unclear so far whether the duller and brighter M^+D^+ cells are part of a single maturation sequence and, if so, which ones are the more mature.

3.   T cells in old mice

Data obtained with immunofluorescence microscopy for nine 28 to 30 month-old CBA mice and the same number of three-month-old controls are summarized in Table 3.

TABLE 3 - FREQUENCY OF CELLS CARRYING T AND B CELL MARKERS IN 9 YOUNG ADULT (3-MONTH-OLD) AND 9 OLD (28 TO 30-MONTH-OLD) MALE CBA/Ca MICE

| Organ | Age | Percentage of cells positive for | | | | Ratio |
		Thy-1	Lyt-1	Lyt-2	sIg	Lyt-2/Thy-1
Spleen	young	27-36	24-41	9-18	35-64	0.29 - 0.50
	old	16-44	13-39	5-17	37-80	0.24 - 0.66
Thymus	young	93-100	73-91	80-93	0- 1	0.79 - 0.98
	old*	73- 86	66-92	55-80	0-22	0.64 - 1.00
Lymph	young	50-76	54-85	23-33	18-33	0.37 - 0.50
nodes	old	44-68	52-68	30-39	31-47	0.54 - 0.79

*Data based on 8 animals only. The ninth animal was omitted from the Table because it had only 12% Thy-1$^+$ cells in its thymus.

The data emphasize the considerable variability between individuals which is commonly seen in old animals. However, there was a clear trend towards reduction in the frequency of Thy-1$^+$ cells in spleen, lymph nodes and thymus. Concomitantly, the frequency of sIg$^+$ cells tended to rise. The relative frequency of Lyt-2$^+$ cells was markedly raised in the old lymph nodes. It should be noted that the brightness of staining with anti-Lyt-1 is heterogeneous and in some cells scarcely above background (Ledbetter et al., 1980). Thus microscopic examination, in particular, is liable to underestimate the frequency of Lyt-1$^+$ cells. This probably accounts for the fact that estimates for Lyt-1$^+$ were often slightly lower than for Thy-1$^+$ in this series of observations.

TABLE 4 - FREQUENCY OF THY-1 AND LYT-2 POSITIVE CELLS IN PERIPHERAL BLOOD
OF CBA/Ca, (BALB/c x SJL/J)F1 AND CBA/Rij MICE

Strain	Age	N	Thy-1	Lyt-2	Lyt-2/Thy 1
CBA/Ca	young*	8	35-50	7-14	0.20 - 0.29
male	middle	5	40-59	10-14	0.24 - 0.28
	old	5	24-33	8-19	0.27 - 0.76
(BALB/c x	young	8	50-69	9-21	0.16 - 0.38
SJL/J)F1	middle	10	18-60	6-16	0.23 - 0.33
female	old	18	12-92	1-82	0.07 - 0.91
(BALB/c x	young	12	52-69	13-21	0.23 - 0.33
SJL/J)F1	middle	16	13-52	4-17	0.25 - 0.42
male	old		n.d.	n.d.	n.d.
CBA/Rij**	young	10	29-58	8-12	0.17 - 0.28
male	middle	9	14-44	5-13	0.26 - 0.36
	old	8	10-34	6-27	0.50 - 0.79

* young = 3 to 4-month old; middle = 10 to 14-month-old; old = 24 to 30-month-old.

**bred at the Institute for Experimental Gerontology TNO, Rijswijk, The Netherlands.

Table 4 summarizes FACS analyses of peripheral blood lymphocyte samples obtained from series of ageing CBA and (BALB/c × SJL/J)F1 mice. Again Lyt-2[+] cells tended to become more frequent in relation to the total Thy-1[+] population as the mice aged. In contrast to Brennan and Jaroslow (1975) we did not observe age-related changes in the density of Thy-1 as measured with the FACS.

DISCUSSION

The introduction of the Lyt-1, 2 and 3 antigens as markers for T cell subpopulations constituted one of the major advances in cellular immunology. Although it is now apparent that Lyt-1 is on more adult T cells and Lyt-2 is on fewer that originally thought, the practical utility of the Lyt antigens as functional subpopulation markers remains undiminished. In fact, the use of monoclonal anti-Lyt antibodies and FACS analysis broadens the basis for subpopulation definition, allowing quantitative as well as qualitative criteria to be used in relating antigen expression to cell subsets.

On the basis of these criteria, we conclude that the subset composition of splenic T cells at 10-14 days of age is similar to that in adults. This does not agree with the report (Cantor & Boyse, 1975a) that over 80% of T cells in spleens of that age were killed by either anti-Lyt-1 or anti-Lyt-2 and complement, and were therefore Lyt-1+,2[+] and presumed to be a predominantly immature population.

The reasons for this disparity remain unclear but could possibly involve the presence of contaminating antibodies in the conventional antisera previously used. Cantor & Boyse (1975a) also found a much higher frequency of nucleated spleen cells carrying Lyt-1 and/or Lyt-2 at 1-2 weeks of age than we do in this report; this again may be attributable to contaminating antibodies, although differences in the extend of splenic erythropoiesis present maybe another explanation. Like Raff & Owen (1971) we have found a near adult T cell frequency in mesenteric lymph nodes at one week of age, and here erythropoiesis is unlikely to be present.

Alternatively, the C57BL/6J strain used by Cantor and Boyse may be exceptionally high in Lyt-2 over Thy-1. Suggestive data in this direction have been presented by Raulet et al., 1980. In a limited survey of the strains available at Rijswijk (comprising among others C57BL/Ka and

C57BL/Rij, but not C57BL/6J) we were unable to verify this particularity of the C57BL strain.

In contrast to the spleen, the Thy-1 and Lyt-1 staining profiles of thymus was approaching the adult pattern by four days of age - that is, a subpopulation with the staining characteristics of medullary thymocytes and peripheral T cells had made its appearance. This subpopulation was therefore available to colonize peripheral lymphoid tissues, although it remains uncertain whether it actually does so or whether, on the contrary, both the medullary thymocytes and peripheral T cells arise independently from cortical thymocytes. The latter alternative would be in line with one of the current views on the origin of T cells in adults (Weissman et al., 1975; Stutman, 1977).

B cells appear to differentiate from pre-B cells which contain μ chains in their cytoplasm (Raff et al., 1976). Along this differentiation pathway there is most likely a stage in which surface IgM is expressed, but not surface IgD.

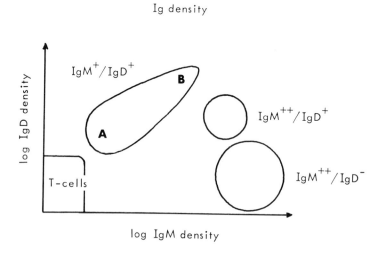

B - cell subpopulations
Ig density

Fig 3. Schematic representation of sIgM and sIgD on developing B-cells

This follows from two observations: 1) most B cells in bone marrow express IgM but not IgD; 2) the first SIg positive cells during ontogeny in the spleen are $M^{++}D^-$ (Scher et al., 1976). Originally it was thought that IgD would be gained by the maturing B-lymphocyte as the IgM was gradually lost (Goding et al., 1977). Our data showing a positive, instead of a negative correlation between the density of sIgM and sIgD (see Fig. 3 for a schematic representation of the various B cell subpopulations as defined by sIgM and sIgD densities) render this mechanism unlikely and suggest two alternatives: 1) in the process of losing sIgM the B lymphocyte aquires first a high density of sIgD and subsequently sIgM and sIgD are lost from the membrane; 2) the $M^+ + D^-$ immature B cell first loses its sIgM and then reaquires it together with sIgD. Proof for either alternative is lacking. However, the second alternative would be more in line with the supposed co-transcription of μ and δ genes from the DNA (for a review, see Gottlieb, 1980), but raises the question whether the sIgM from $M^{++}D^-$ cells and that of M^+D^+ is coded for by the same gene. It should be noted that the existence of the $M^{++}D^+$ cell argues against our alternative number 2.

The lymph nodes and peripheral blood of old mice show a clear tendency for the proportion of T cells which are $Lyt-2^+$ and probably, although we have few data, $Lyt-3^+$ (Lyt-2 and 3 are on the same molecule; Ledbetter & Herzenberg, 1979) to increase. This is less evident in the spleen, but there may be no real difference. There have been several reports of high suppressor cell activity in old mice, possibly accounting for the low responses often observed to various antigens (Goidl et al., 1976; Segre and Segre, 1976; Krogsrud and Perkins, 1977; Makinodan, 1980) and T suppressor cells are $Lyt-2^+$ (Cantor et al., 1976; Beverly et al., 1976). The ratio of T to B cells tended to decrease in old mice, so that in absolute terms there was a loss of $Lyt-1+,2^-$ (helper ?) cells rather than an increase of suppressors. Thus the balance between help and suppression may have been upset in the older animals.

ACKNOWLEDGEMENTS

Many of the experiments reported here were performed at the Department of Genetics, Stanford University School of Medicine. We are particularly indebted to Drs. Len and Lee Herzenberg and Jeffrey Ledbetter and to Mr. Jeffrey Dangl and Mr. Eugene Filson, for their collaboration and help. J.J.Haaijman was in receipt of an Arthritis Foundation Fellowship and H.S. Micklem of a travel grant from the Wellcome Trust. This work was supported in part by grants from the National Institutes of Health (CA-04681 and GM-17367) and the U.K. Medical Research Council.

REFERENCES

Abney, E.R., Cooper, M.D., Kearney, J.F., Lawton, A.R., and Parkhouse, R.M.E., 1978. Sequential expression of immunoglobulin on developing mouse B lymphocytes: a systematic survey that suggests a model for the generation of immunoglobulin isotype diversity. J.Immunol. 120: 2041.

Bayer, E.A., and Wilchek, M., 1974. Insolubilized biotin for the purification of avidin. Methods in Enzymol. 34: 265.

Beverly, P.C.L., Woody, J., Dunkley, M., Feldmann, M., and McKenzie, I., 1976. Separation of suppressor and killer T cells by surface phenotype. Nature, 262: 495.

Brennan, P.C., and Jaroslow, B.N., 1975. Age-associated decline in theta antigen on spleen thymus-derived lymphocytes of B6CF1 mice. Cell Immunol., 15: 51.

Cantor, H., and Boyse, E.A., 1975a. Functional subclasses of T lymphocytes bearing different Ly antigens. I, The generation of functionally distinct T-cell subclasses in a differentiative process independent of antigen. J.Exp.Med., 141: 1376.

Cantor, H., and Boyse, E.A., 1976b. Functional subclasses of T lymphocyte bearing different Ly antigens. II, Cooperation between subclasses of Ly^4 cells in the generation of killer activity. J.Exp.Med., 141: 1390.

Cantor, H., Shen, F.W., and Boyse, E.A., 1976. Separation of helper T cells from suppressor T cells expressing different Ly components. II. Activation by antigen: after immunization, antigen-specific suppressor and helper activities are mediated by distinct T-cell subclasses. J.Exp.Med., 143: 1391.

Eckhardt, L.A., and Herzenberg, L.A., 1980. Monoclonal antibodies to ThB detect close linkage of Ly-6 and a gene regulating ThB expression. Immunogenetics, 11: 275.

Goding, J.W., Scott, D.W., and Layton, J.E., 1977. Genetics, cellular expression and function of IgD and IgM receptors. Immunol.Rev., 37: 152.

Goidl, E.A., Innes, J.B., and Weksler, M.E., 1976. Immunological studies of aging. II. Loss of IgG and high avidity plague-forming cells and increased suppressor cell activity in aging mice. J.Exp.Med., 144: 1037.

Gottlieb, P.D., 1980. Immunoglobulins genes. Molecular Immunol., 17: 1423.

Haaijman, J.J., 1981. Production of monoclonal antibodies for the analysis of the ontogeny of the murine lymphoid system with flow fluorometry. In: G.Wick (Ed.) Advanced immunofluorescence. in the press.

Haaijman, J.J., Micklem, H.S., Ledbetter, J.A., Dangl, J.L., Herzenberg, L.A.,and Herzenberg, L.A., 1981. T cell ontogeny: organ location of maturing populations (defined by surface antigen markers) is similar in neonates and adults. J.Exp.Med. 153: 605.

Herzenberg, L.A., and Herzenberg, L.A., 1978. !n: D.M. Weir (Ed.) Handbook of Experimental Immunology, 3rd edition, Blackwell Scientific Publications, Oxford. Chapter 22.

Krogsrud, R., and Perkins, E.H., 1977. Age-related changes in T cell function. J.Immunol., 118: 1607.

Ledbetter, J.A., and Herzenberg, L.A., 1979. Xenogenic monoclonal antibodies to mouse lymphoid differentiation antigens. Immunol.Rev., 47: 63.

Ledbetter, J.A. Rouse, R.V., Micklem, H.S., and Herzenberg, L.A., 1980. T cell subsets defined by expression of Lyt-1,2,3 and Thy-1 antigens. J.Exp.Med., 152: 280.

Makinodan, T., 1980. Nature of the decline in antigen-induced humoral immunity with age. Mech.Ageing Develop., 14: 165.

Oi, V.T., Jones, P.P., Goding, J.W., Herzenberg, L.A., and Herzenberg, L.A., 1978. Properties of monoclonal antibodies to mouse Ig allotypes, H-2 and Ia antigens. Curr.Topics Microbiol.Immunol., 81: 115.

Potter, T.A., Hogarth, P.M., and McKenzie, I., 1980. Flow microfluorometric analysis of alloantigen expression during T cell development. Eur.J.Immunol., 10: 899.

Raff, M.C., and Owen, J.T.T., 1971. Thymus-derived lymphocytes: their distribution and role in the development of peripheral lymphoid tissues of the mouse. Eur.J.Immunol., 1: 27.

Raff, M.C., Megson, M., Owen, J.J.T., and Cooper, M.D., 1976. Early production of intracellular IgM by B lymphocyte precursors in mouse. Nature, 259: 224.

Raulet, D.H., Gottlieb, P.D., and Bevan, M.J., 1980. Fractionation of lymphocyte populations with monoclonal antibodies specific for Lyt-2.2 and Lyt-3.1. J.Immunol., 125: 1136.

Scher, I., Berning, A.K., Kessler, S., and Finkelman, F.D., 1980. Development of B lymphocytes in the mouse; studies of the frequency and distribution of surface IgM and IgD in normal and immune-defective CBA/N F1 mice. J.Immunol., 125: 1686.

Segre, D., and Segre, M., 1976. Humoral immunity in aged mice. II. Increased suppressor T cell activity in immunologically deficient old mice. J.Immunol., 116: 735.

Shiku, H., Kisielow, P., Bean, M.A., Takahashi, T., Boyse, E.A., Oettgen, H.E., and Old, L.J., 1975. Expression of T cell differentiation antigens on effector cells in cell-mediated cytoxicity in vitro. J.Exp.Med., 141: 227.

Stutman, O., 1977. Two main features of T-cell development: thymus traffic and post thymic maturation. Contemp. Topics in Immunobiology, 7: 1.

Vitetta, E.S., Melcher, U., McWilliams, M., Lamm, M.E., Phillips-Quagliata, J.M., and Uhr, J.W., 1975. Cell surface immunoglobulin. XI. The appearance of an IgD-like molecule on murine lymphoid cells during ontogeny. J.Exp.Med., 141: 206.

Weissman, I.L., Masuda, T., Olive, C., and Friedberg, S.H., 1975. Differentiation and migration of T lymphocytes. Israel J.Med.Sci., 11: 1267.

Wysocki, L.J., and Sato, V.L., 1978. 'Panning' for lymphocytes: a method for cell selection. Proc.Natl.Acad.Sci. USA, 75: 2844.

EFFECT OF AGEING AND ADULT THYMECTOMY (A-Tx) ON PRIMARY SYNGE-
NEIC SENSITIZATION ON MONOLAYERS OF THYROID EPITHELIAL CELLS
(TEC)

Jeannine Charreire

INSERM U 25 - Hôpital Necker

161, rue de Sèvres - 75015 Paris - France

ABSTRACT

Using an in vitro model of sensitization of lymphoid T
cells on monolayers of syngeneic thyroid epithelial cells,
previously developed by us , we studied the role of ageing
and adult thymectomy (which can be considered as an accelerated process of ageing). We demonstrated that the thymus,
spleen and bone marrow of normal animals, show optimal syngeneic sensitization by three months of age, a significant
decrease being found with ageing after that time. Conversely,
syngeneic sensitization with lymph node cells increases with
age, the highest values being found when animals were eighteen
months old.
Adult thymectomy induces as early as 7 days and until
three months following surgery an increase in thymidine upta -
ke by lymph node cells. Then, this phenomenon is abrogated and
normal values are recovered. Bone marrow cells of such animals behave like controls until three months after adult thymectomy and suddenly drop off. In contrast, their spleen cells
show a transient decrease until three months after surgery
followed by an increase of syngeneic sensitization.
All these results suggest that ageing or adult thymectomy
is accompanied by a loss of suppressor cells, mainly among
lymph node cells.

INTRODUCTION

The immune system does not normally react to "self" anti-

gens. However, under certain circumstances, such as thymus

deprivation (Charreire and Bach, 1975 ; Carnaud et al.,1977)

polyclonal stimulation (Hammarström et al.,1976) drug indu-

ced selective depletion of lymphoid cell elements (L'Age Stehr

and Diamanstein, 1978) stimulation by syngeneic tissue anti-

gens modified by the presence of a virus (Doherty et al.,1976)

or a chemical hapten (Shearer et al.,1976), thymocytes may

become reactive to syngeneic or autologous stimuli. Such situ-

ations are found in newborn (Small et al.,1975) or adult

thymectomy (ATx) (Charreire and Bach, 1975) and in ageing subjects (Fournier and Charreire, 1977, Fournier and Charreire,
in press ; Gozes et al., 1978).

Recently, we have developed an in vitro model of syngeneic sensitization on thyroid epithelial cells (TEC) in
which we demonstrated that sensitization is specifically directed against structures born by syngeneic thyroid cells
only (Yeni and Charreire, in press). Moreover, we show that
sensitized lymphocytes belong to the T cell lineage (Charreire, submitted for publication) and are responsible for the
induction of thyroiditis when transferred into syngeneic intact recipients (Charreire and Michel-Bechet, submitted for
publication).

The aim of this report is the study of the effect of
ageing and ATx on primary syngeneic sensitization on monolayers of TEC.

MATERIALS AND METHODS

1/ Animals - Lymphoid cells were obtained from 7 day to 18-
month-old CBA ($H-2^k$) strain of mice. Thyroids were collected
from 3 to 5-month-old CBA mice. All animals were purchased
from the C.S.E.A.L., C.N.R.S. Orléans La Source, France.
Thymectomy of adult mice (3 months) was performed using the
suction technique described by J.F.A.P. Miller.

2/ Mouse thyroid cell culture - Thyroid cultures were performed according to a technique previously described (Yeni et
al., 1980). Thyroids were carefully dissected and minced
with scissors into small pieces at 4°C in RPMI 1640 containing
50 µg/ml penicillin, 50 µg/ml streptomycin and 2.5. µg/ml
fungizone (complete medium). The suspension was then incubated
with 1.5 mg/ml collagenase (Boehringer-Mannheim, Western Germany) in a shaking water bath at 37°C for 30 min. After centrifugation (10 min, 250 g) a second treatment with fresh
collagenase medium was performed as described above. The enzymatic secretion was stopped by incubation of the thyroid cells
for 5 min in complete medium plus 20% fetal calf serum (FCS)

and centrifuged at 150 g for 7 min. Then, the pellet containing viable single thyroid cells and complete follicules was
resuspended before cell counting. About 2×10^4 cells in
0.2 ml were incubated in a flat bottomed Microtest II (Falcon
n°3042) tissue culture dish. Incubation was performed in a
humidified atmosphere of 5% CO_2 in air. The culture medium
was changed twice a week. After 10 to 12 days of incubation,
a confluent monolayer was obtained and used for primary sensitization.

3/ Cell cultures- Lymphoid cell suspensions in complete RPMI
medium without sera, because of their blocking effect (Yeni and
Charreire, in press) were settled on confluent monolayers of syngeneic thyroid cells. In any case, for each population, three
concentrations of cells were sensitized :0.12, 0.25 and 0.50 x
10^6 cells per well in 0.2 ml. Identical concentrations of
lymphoid cells were cultured alone without any sensitization
in order to determine the spontaneous thymidine incorporation
of lymphocytes. Under normal conditions, cultures were performed in flat bottomed microplates (Falcon 3020) and cultured
in 5% CO_2 in a humidified incubator for 72 hours. After 60
hours of culture, 1 µCi of ^{3}H thymidine (specific activity
1 µCi per millimole) was added. The cells were then harvested
with a multiple automated sample harvester, and the radioactivity incorporated by the cells was determined by liquid
scintillation counting. In all cases, cultures were performed
in triplicates. The results were expressed as mean cpm of
thymidine incorporation in triplicates of sensitized lymphocytes minus mean cpm of thymidine incorporation or triplicates
of control lymphocytes alone.

4/ Statistical analysis was carried out using the Student'
"t" test.

RESULTS

1/ Effect of ageing of primary sensitization on syngeneic monolayers of TEC

Lymphocytes obtained from spleen, lymph nodes, thymus and bone marrow of intact CBA donors aged from 7 days to 18 months, were cultured for 3 days either on syngeneic monolayers of TEC, or alone as controls, and the specific thymidine uptake calculated as described above. In most of the experiments, the optimal specific thymidine incorporation occurs when 0.25×10^6 cells per well were co-cultured. Results are shown on Fig.1.

FIGURE 1 - Effect of ageing on syngeneic sensitization on monolayers of TEC of lymphoid organs of CBA mice. Mean $\pm$ S.E.M. of 3 experiments - 0.25×10^6 cells per well

●----● bone marrow   O——o   lymph node

■----■ spleen   △·-·-·△   thymus

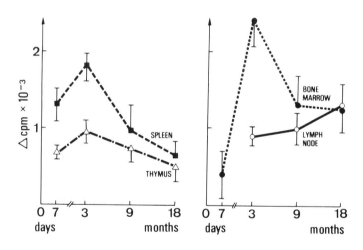

Syngeneic sensitization obtained with thymus from animals 8 days, 3 months, 9 months or 18 months old remains at a low level and never exceeds 1000cpm. Spleen cells exhibit as early as 7 days after birth a thymidine uptake inferior to the optimal values obtained at 3 months of age. On 9,and mainly on 18-month-old spleen cells, a diminution of specific syngeneic sensitization of respectively 40% and 60% is observed.

Syngeneic sensitization seen with bone marrow cells of animals of different ages shows a pattern similar to that of spleen cells. However, thymidine uptake, demonstrated with bone marrow cells from 7-day-old animals is lower, compared to that obtained from 3-month-old donors. Then, when animals are 9 or 18 months old, the syngeneic sensitization of their bone marrow cells remains depressed.

The syngeneic sensitization was also studied using lymph node cells from animals aged   3,9 and 18 months. It was not possible to study lymph nodes from 8-day-old animals because of their small size. As shown on Fig.1, thymidine uptake by lymph node cells increases with age, but always remains at a level inferior to those found with spleen or bone marrow cells of 3-month-old animals.

2/ Effect of adult thymectomy on primary sensitization on syngeneic monolayers of TEC

Lymphoid organs from mice ATxed 7 days, 1 month, 3 months or more than 6 months, prior to usage, were co-cultured with monolayers of syngeneic TEC. As shown on Fig.2, thymidine uptake by spleen cells from ATx animals, 7 days following surgery, behave like spleen cells of normal controls. In contrast, a 20% and a 50% decrease was found with spleen cells from animals respectively thymectomized for 1 and 3 months. This diminution seems to be a transient phenomenon since, when similar co-cultures were performed with spleen cells provided by those animals thymectomized for at least 6 months, a level of thymidine uptake similar to that of sham-operated controls was noted.

FIGURE 2 - Effect of adult thymectomy on syngeneic sensitiza-
tion on monolayers of TEC of lymphoid organs of
CBA mice at different times after surgery. Mean ±
S.E.M. of 4 to 7 experiments. 0.25 x 10^6 cells/well

●---● bone marrow   o——o lymph node   ■——■ spleen

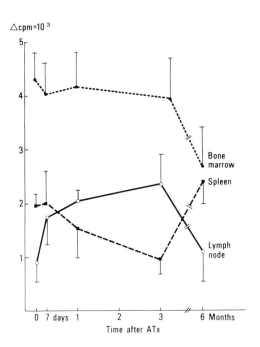

Syngeneic stimulation induced by co)cultures of lymph
node cells from ATxed mice shows a different curve. In the
initial period, an increase of 60% by day 7, 100% by one
month, and 120% by 3 months following ATx is observed. Then,
at least 6 months after surgery, a decrease in syngeneic sensitization is found, leading to values identical to those of
sham-operated control mice.

Syngeneic sensitization of bone marrow cells, 7 days,
1 month, or 3 months after surgery, never exhibits any modifications. However, 6 months after ATx a 30% decrease in thymidine incorporation is regularly found.

DISCUSSION

Our previous data (Yeni et al., 1980) indicate that normal T cells incorporate thymidine after previous contact with syngeneic thyroid monolayers. We have shown that this response is specific to syngeneic thyroid since it is suppressed by depletion of lymphocytes binding to thyroid cells and it is specifically enhanced by a secondary exposure to syngeneic thyroid monolayers (Yeni and Charreire,in press).. We also demonstrated that thyroid-sensitized lymphoblasts, and more precisely T lymphoblasts, are able to induce thyroiditis when injected into syngeneic recipients (Charreire et Michel-Bechet, submitted for publication).

The effects of ATx and ageing can be compared to those found in mice 48 hours after injection of 20 mg/kg of cyclo-phosphamide (Charreire, submitted to publication). In this instance, syngeneic sensitization was diminished in the spleen, the thymus and the bone marrow of the recipients, while lymph node cells showed a significant augmentation of thymidine up-take. It can be assumed that ATx or ageing act by two diffe-rent mechanisms : first, a T cell depletion of cyclophospha-mide-sensitive suppressor cells, mainly located in the lymph nodes of normal recipients (Dutton, 1975), and second, a diminution, mainly in ATxed animals, of short-lived self-reacti-ve T cells. The increase of syngeneic sensitization of CBA spleen cells 6 months after ATx is in agreement with our previous data on autorosette-forming cells (Charreire and Bach, 1975) and with those of Droege (1979) on TNP modified syngeneic cytotoxicity.

The role of T cells in self-recognition has been well documented in various in vitro models : syngeneic sensitiza-tion on fibroblasts or thymus cells (Cohen and Wekerle,1972) or autologous testis cells (Wekerle, 1978), binding of lympho-cytes to autologous or syngeneic red blood cells in mice (Charreire and Bach,1974) or in humans (Fournier and Charrei-re, 1977) and as responder cells in autologous MLR in mice

(Boehmer and Von Byrd, 1972) or in humans (Kuntz et al., 1976 Fournier and Charreire, in press). All these data, considered with this in vitro model of primary syngeneic sensitization on monolayers of TEC, strongly demonstrate a predominant role of T cells in self-recognition, and more precisely in the induction of thyroiditis (Charreire and Michel-Bechet, submitted for publication). These results concerning the effect of ageing and ATx in the sensitization on syngeneic TEC further strengthen the hypothesis of T cell involvement in self recognition.

ACKNOWLEDGMENTS

We thank Miss E. LALLEMAND for her skillful technical help and Miss J. JACOBSON for her invaluable editorial assistance.

108

REFERENCES

Boehmer,H. von and Byrd,W.J. (1972) Responsiveness of
thymus cells to syngeneic and allogeneic lymphoid cells.
Nature, New Biology, 235, 50-52.

Carnaud,C., Charreire, J. and Bach,J.F. (1977) Adult thymectomy promotes the manifestion of autoreactive lymphocytes. Cell.Immunol. 28 , 274-283.

Charreire, J. and Bach,J.F. (1974) Self and non self.
Lancet, 2, 229.

Charreire, J. and Bach,J.F. (1975) Binding of autologous
erythrocytes to immature T cells. Proc.Natl.Acad.Sci.
USA, 72 , 2301-3205.

Charreire, J. Syngeneic sensitization of mouse lymphocytes on monolayers of thyroid epithelial cells. II.
T and B cell involvement in primary response
(submitted for publication).

Charreire, J. and Michel-Bechet,M. Syngeneic sensitization
of mouse lymphocytes on monolayers of thyroid epithelial cells. III. Induction of thyroiditis by thyroid
sensitized T lymphoblasts (submitted for publication).

Cohen,I.R. and Wekerle,H. (1972) Autosensitization of
lymphocytes against thymus reticulum cells. Science,
176, 1324-1325.

Doherty,P.C., Blanden,R.V. and Zinkernagel,R.M. (1976)
Specificity of virus immune effector T cells for H-2K
or H-2D compatible interactions : implications for
H-diversity. Transplant.Rev. 29 , 89-124.

Droege ,W., Suessmuth,W., Franze,R., Mueller,P., Franze,W.
and Balcarova,J. (1979) Suppressor cells regulating the
in vivo induction of cytotoxic T lymphocytes and of
memory cells for a secondary in vitro CMC response.
in " Cell Biology and Immunology of Leucocyte Function"
ed. M.R.Quastel, pp. 467-483 (Academic Press New YOrk).

Dutton,R.W. (1975) Suppressor T cells. Transpl.Rev. 26,
39-55.

Fournier, C. and Charreire,J.(1977) Increase in autologous
erythrocyte binding by T cells with ageing in man.
Clin.Exp.Immunol., 29, 468-473.

Fournier,C. and Charreire,J. Autologous mixed lymphocyte
reaction in man. I. Relationship with age and sex.
Cell.Immunol. (in press).

Gozes,Y., Umiel,T., Meshorer,A. and Trainin,N. (1978)
Syngenenic GVH induced in popliteal lymph nodes by
spleen cells of old C57BL/6 mice. J.Immunol.,121,
2199-2204.

Hammarström,L., Smith,E., Primi,D. and Möller,G. (1976) Induction of antibody response to autologous red blood cells in bovine spleen cells by polyclonal B cell activators. Nature, London, 263, 60-63.

Kuntz,N.N., Innes,J..B., and Weksler,M.E. (1976) Lymphocyte transformation induced by autologous cells. IV. Human T lymphocyte proliferation induced by autologous or allogeneic non T cell lymphocytes. J.Exp.Med. 143, 1042-1054.

L'Age-Stehr,J. and Diamanstein,T. Induction of autoreactive T lymphocytes and their suppressor cells by cyclophosphamide. (1978) Nature, London, 271, 663-665.

Shaerer,G.M., Rehn,T.G. and Schmitt-Verhulst,A.M. (1976). Role of the murine major histocompatibility complex in the specificity of in vitro T cell mediated lympholysis against chemically modified autologous lymphocytes. Transpl.Rev. 29 , 222-246.

Small,M.,and Trainin,N. (1975) Control of autoreactivity by a humoral factor of the thymus (THF). Cell.Immunol. 20 , 1-11.

Wekerle,H. (1978) Immunological T cell memory in the in vitro induced experimental autoimmune orchitis. Specificity of the reaction and tissue distribution of the autoantigens. J.Exp.Med. 147, 233-250.

Yeni,P., Michel-Bechet,M., Athonel-Haou,A.M., Fayet,G. and Charreire,J. (1980) In vitro induction of immunological memory against epithelial cells of thyroid origin in mice. in "Autoimmune Aspects of Endocrine disorders" A.Pinchera, D.Doniach, G.F.Fenzi and L.Baschieri,eds. pp.207-213, Academic Press, London.

Yeni,P. and Charreire,J. Syngeneic sensitization of mouse lymphocytes on monolayers of thyroid epithelial cells. I. Study of proliferative response. Cell.Immunol. (in press).

-:-:-:-

INCREASED OCCURRENCE OF SELF REACTIVE T CELL CLONES IN THE AGING IMMUNE SYSTEM

Helga Schneider and Hartmut Wekerle

Max-Planck-Institut für Immunbiologie, Stübeweg 51,

Freiburg i.Br., FRG

ABSTRACT

Studies in our laboratory have indicated that in senescent rats there is a paradoxical increase of T cell self reactivity, when T cell reactivity against foreign antigenic determinants is declining. These investigations were performed by determining T cell dependent cytostatic activity of bulk cultures. This increased autoreactivity may have been brought about by an increased presence of potentially self reactive clones or by a defect in intercellular regulation. To test this we cultured rat T lymphocytes with an excess of syngeneic stimulator cells and estimated the proportion of self reactive T cells with a limiting dilution assay. In young rats the number of self reactive T cells was 1/15.000 by 24 months of age this rate had increased to 1/7.000. The proportion of alloreactive T cells remained constant over a wide range of age, did not change rapidly with age and showed a declining tendency only very late in life.

INTRODUCTION

Kyewski and Wekerle (1978) demonstrated in experimental autoimmune orchitis that autoreactivity, determined by the cytostasis assay, was significantly higher in aging inbred rats (< 19 months) than in animals aged from 3 to 5 months. There is also some evidence derived from bulk proliferation cultures that self reactivity in older rats is enhanced compared to younger ones. In bulk cultures and in experimental autoimmune orchitis the augmented self reactivity could be ascribed to T lymphocytes. It is not known whether loss of self tolerance with increasing age results from a decline in regulator cell control or is due to dysfunction of T helper cells or a combination (Goidl et al., 1976, Kay, 1978, Krogsrud andPerkins, 1977).

MATERIALS AND METHODS

Rats: Young (3 months of age) and aging rats of different strains (23 to 33 months), were obtained from the Institute für experimental Gerontology TNO, Rijswijk, The Netherlands, and from the breeding facilities of the MPI in Freiburg, Germany.

Limiting dilution culture: Lymph node lymphocytes (responder cells) were cultured with syngeneic stimulator cells, which had been irridiated with 2.000 R. It is known that the stimulator cells (antigen) resemble reticulum cells whereas responder cells are T cells. The responder cells were added in dilutions from 24.000 to 700 to 1×10^6 stimulator cells per well. The culture medium (Dulbecco's modified Eagle's medium, GIBCO, G and Island, N.Y.) was supplemented with 15% horse serum (GIBCO) and 0.05 mM 2-mercaptoethanol. To ensure adequate contact, cultures were initially set up in V-bottomed microtiter plates (Greiner, Nürtingen, Germany) and transferred to round bottom microtiter plates two days later (Nune, Reskilde, Denmark). Twelve replicate cultures for each dilution were set up and the cultures were read as positive or negative after 10 days. The precursor frequencies in limiting dilution cultures were calculated from the knowledge that the relationship between the percentage of nonresponding cultures per group and the number of responding cells per microculture obeys a Poisson distribution; by definition there is one precursor cell per well if 37% of the wells are negative (Ryser and MacDonald, 1979; Corley et al., 1978).

RESULTS

Employing a limiting dilution assay we found that self reactivity in aging rats (< 24 months) is enhanced compared to young controls (3 to 5 months), whereas the alloreactivity declines when the rats are older than 29 months. An example of the autoreactivity in MLCs of young and old rats are given in Fig. 1. The frequency at 37% negative reacting cultures for 24 months old Lewis rats was 1/6.200 and 1/7.200 whereas the frequency for younger animals was only 1/23.000 and less than 1/25.000. We also compared autologous and syngeneic combinations because it appeared possible that within the 2 year interval spaning both generation genetic fluctuations could have occurred, although all the rat strains employed are known to be highly inbred. The respondsiveness of aging lymphocytes against young and aging stimulator cells was tested and, in parallel, the responsiveness of young lymphocytes against both types of stimulator cells. The increased precursor frequencies of the older rats were solely due to aged T lymphocytes and there was no difference in the autoantigenicity of both types of stimulator cells. In the allogeneic MLC the outcome was the opposite, but the tendency was not so clear cut with the syngeneic MLC. In the latter case the precursor frequency showed a significant increase after 24 months, whereas the proportion of alloreactive T cells remained constant over a wide range declined onl in late stages of life (< 29 months), Fig. 2. Because the precursor frequencies in allogeneic MLCs were relatively low, we tried to augment the alloreactivity either with syngeneic helper cells or with pure allogeneic stimulator cells (in most cases we tested MHC

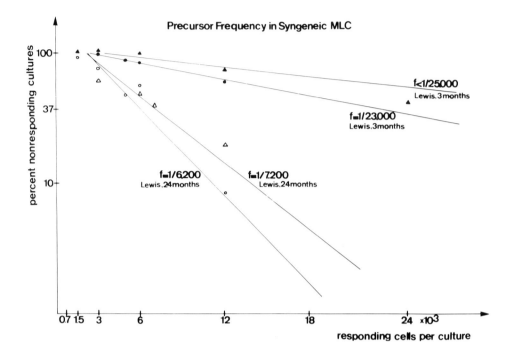

Fig. 1

PRECURSOR FREQUENCIES IN SYNGENEIC MLC OF 24 MONTHS OLD INBRED
LEWIS RATS AND THE YOUNG CONTROLS (3 TO 5 MONTHS).
On the ordinate, the percentage of negative reacting cultures is marked, on the
abscissa the number of responder cells per well is listed.
The concentration of syngeneic stimulator cells was 1×10^6 per well. The cultures
were read at day ten.

congenic combinations). The helper cells used were either lymph node lymphocytes,
spleen cells or thymocytes. No increase was observed. There were also no changes
in the precursor frequencies independent of whether we used MHC congeneic or
pure allogeneic stimulator cells.

CONCLUSIONS

There are two basic mechanisms which may underlie self tolerance: firstly
a state of central nonreactivity which is due to an irreversible loss of self-reactive, competent lymphocytes; secondly a state of peripheral inhibition in which
potential self reactive lymphocytes exist, but are suppressed or not stimulated. The
first concept is compatible with Burnet's clonal selection theory (Burnet, 1949).

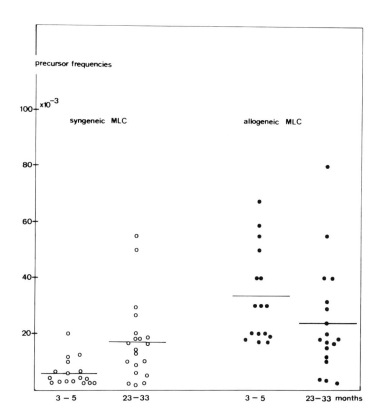

Fig. 2

SUMMARY OF PRECURSOR FREQUENCIES IN SYNGENEIC AND ALLOGENEIC
MLC.
The controls (3 to 5 months) are on the left, the data of the old rats (> 24 months)
are on the right. In the syngeneic reaction the frequencies of precursor cells are
significantly increased compared to the controls ($p < 0.002$). In the allogeneic
reaction the frequencies of precursor cells were decreased compared to the young
rats ($p < 0.01$).

The second concept takes into account that the immune system may consist of a
network of complicated regulation mechanisms between lymphocyte subpopulations; here the phenomenon of selfrecognition is of basic importance (Cohen and
Wekerle, 1977). Autoreactivity represents an interaction between self-reactive
lymphocytes and peripheral cells from the same organism. This interaction with
presumes specific selfrecognition should not be regarded per se as pathological, but
seems to be a prerequisite for the total intercellular communication. Such

processes seem to be operating during differentiation and in the adult organism, especially between cellular components of the immune system (Cantor, 1978; Wigzell, 1977; Köhler and Rowley, 1977). This loss in the ability to discriminate between self and nonself may have its root in pathological changes as follows: a) the appearence of new, so-called autoaggressive, forbidden clones (Profitt et al., 1977) or may be due to a defect in the control of such clones existing in vivo (Cantor, 1978) which leads to a general autoimmune tendency; b) structural changes in organ specific autoantigens or contact of the immune system with sequestered antigens which are not self tolerated (Barker and Billingham, 1977).

The immune system of the aging organism is marked by a general loss of T and B cell competence and by an increase in autoimmunity (Walford, 1969). The increase of autoimmunity is linked to a loss of T cell competence in the aged organism (Good and Yunis, 1974; Teague, 1974). It is far from being clear which cellular mechanisms lead to the different manifestations of autoimmunity. This is especially valid for T cell autoreactivity in old age. Is there any analogous increase of autoreactivity at the T cell level, as is known for B cell clones producing autoantibodies, leading to autoimmune diseases in old age ? Kyewski and Wekerle (1978) were able to show with two different in vitro tests (proliferation- and EAO-cytostase-reaction) that in contrast to diminished nonself and mitogen reactivity the reaction of the same, aged lymphocytes against autoantigens is significantly increased. To study whether selfreactivity in old age is due to an increased number of autoreactive clones or due to intercellular defects we employed a limiting dilution assay. Using this assay we found that with increasing age (< 24 months) the number of self reacting T cell clones were increased and that this phenomenon was due to the responding T lymphocytes rather than to stimulator cells. In allogeneic combinations the precursor frequencies decline only in terminal stages of life. This increased precursor frequency seems to be a general feature of aging rats and cannot be a result of a natural selection process, since the animals investigated were taken before they had reached the age of 50% survival, known for these colonies. Because the frequencies remained constant when T helper cells were added we concluded that the helper cells are not altered in the aged organism. The question whether altered suppressor cell activity occurs in old age cannot be answered from our data; although other reports suggest an increase in the number of suppressor cells (De Kruyff et al., 1980; Segre and Segre, 1976).

REFERENCES

Barker, C.F. and Billingham, E.R.: Immunologically Privileged Sites. Adv. Immunol. 25: 1-54, 1977.

Burnet, F.M.: The Clonal Theory of Aquired Immunity. (Cambridge University Press, 1949).

Cantor, H.: Lymphocyte Communication and Autoimmunity. Genetic Control of Autoimmune Disease, Ed. N.R. Rose et al., Vol. 1 pp 151, (Elsevier/North Holland, 1978).

Cohnen ,I.R. and Wekerle, H.: Autoimmunity, Self Recognition and Blocking Factors. Autoimmunity, Ed. N. Talal, pp. 231-266 (Academic Press, 1977).

Corley, R.B.: Kindred, B. and Lefkovits, I.: Positive and Negative Allogeneic Effects Mdiated by MLR-Primed Lymphocytes: Quantitation By Limiting Dilution Analysis. J. Immunol. 121: 1082-1089, 1978.

De Kruyff, R.H., Kimm, Y.T., Siskind, G.W. and Weksler, M.E.: Age Related Changes in the In Vitro Immune Response: Increased Suppressor Activity in Immature and Aged Mice. J. Immunol. 125: 142-147, 1980.

Goidl, E.A., Innes, J.B. and Weksler, M.E.: Immunological Studies of Aging. II. Loss of IgG and High Avidity Plaque-Forming Cells and Increased Suppressor Cell Activity in Aging Mice. J. Exp. Med. 144: 1037-1048, 1976.

Good, R.A. and Yunis, E.J.: Association of Autoimmunity, Immunodeficiency and Aging in Man, Rabbits and Mice. Fed. Proc. 33: 2040-2050, 1974.

Kay, M.M.B.: Effect of Age on T Cell Differentiation. Fed. Proc. 37: 1241-1244, 1978.

Köhler, H. and Rowley, D.A.: Self-recognition: The Basic Principle in the Immune System. Autoimmunity, Ed. N. Talal, pp. 267- (Academic Press, 1977).

Korgsrud, H. and Perkins, E.H.: Age-related Changes in T CEll Function. J. Immunol. 118: 1607-1611, 1977.

Kyewski, B. and Wekerle, H.: Increase of T Lymphocytes Self-reactivity in Aging Inbred Rats: In Vitro Studies With a Model of Experimental Autoimmune Orchitis. J. Immunol. 120: 1249-1255, 1978.

Profitt, M.R., Hirsch, M.S. and Black, P.H.: Viruses, Autoimmunity, and Murine Lymphoma. Autoimmunity, Ed. N. Tala, pp. 395-401 (Academic Press, 1977).

Ryser, J.E. and MacDonald, H.R.: Limiting Dilution Analysis of Alloantigen-reactive T lymphocytes. I. Comarison of Precursor Frequencies for Proliferative and Cytolytic Responses. J. Immunol. 122: 1691-1696, 1979.

Segre, D. an Segre, M.: Humoral Immunity in Aged Mice. II. Increased Suppressor T Cell Activity in Immunologically Deficient Old Mice. J. Immunol. 116: 735-738, 1976.

Teague, P.O.: Spontaneous Autoimmunity and Involution of the Lymphoid System. Fed. Proc. 33: 2051-2052, 1974.

Walford, R.L.: The Immunological Theory of Aging (Munksgaard, Copenhagen, 1969).

Wigzell, H.: Positive Autoimmunity. Autoimmunity, Ed. N. Talal, pp. 693-707, (Academic Press, 1977).

ACKNOWLEDGEMENTS:

We thank Mrs. Rosemary Schneider for typing this manuscript. This work was supported by a grant from the Deutsche Forschungsgemeinschaft.

AGE-RELATED CHANGES IN NUDE SPLEEN CELL FUNCTION

Rita Bösing-Schneider

University of Konstanz, Department of Biology,

Immunology Division, D-7750 Konstanz, West Germany

ABSTRACT

The ability of spleen cells from neonatal and aged nude mice to respond in vitro in the presence of a T cell re-placing factor is reduced. The possible role of suppressor cells in the spleen from older nude mice is studied by trans-ferring memory cells from primed donors to nude mice of different ages. It is shown that memory cells can be activated to give a secondary response only in young nude mice (6 weeks of age). In older mice this capability is impaired. It is concluded that cells from the "prethymic" precursor pool of the nude mouse contribute to this impair-ment.

INTRODUCTION

Extensive studies have been made on lymphocyte differentiation during ontogeny. It has been shown that the delayed onset of the humoral immune response after birth is attributable not only to the absence of mature T-cells but also to immature B-cells (Bösing-Schneider, 1979). Several reports indicate that the magnitude of the humoral immune response is decreased in old mice (Hirokawa and Makinodan, 1975; Segre and Segre, 1976; Makinodan,1978). Since thymus-dependent immune reactions are more severely impaired than thymus-independent immune functions, the in-volution of the thymus gland may be related to this effect. (Weksler et al. 1978). Because the thymus tissue has de-generated in normal aged mice, the thymus-deficient nude mouse might provide us a model of premature aging phe-nomena, with respect to immune function.

MATERIALS AND METHODS

Animals

BALB/c nu/nu mice, derived from our own breeding stock, were used as a source of neonatal, adult and aged spleen cells, deficient in T cells. Donors for normal spleen cells were either BALB/c or BALB-Ig^b of our own breeding stock.

TRF

T-cell replacing factor was produced in spleen cell cultures of normal BALB/c-mice after stimulation by concanavalin A (2 μg/ml); according to the method of Schimpl and Wecker (1972). It was added to spleen cell cultures 24-48 hours after antigenic stimulation.

Cell culture

Spleen cells from neonatal, adult or aged mice were prepared and cultured according to the method of Mishell and Dutton (1967) and incubated in the presence of 2-mercapto-ethanol for 4 days (Click, Benck and Alter, 1972). Sheep red blood cells (SRBC) were used as antigen at a dose of 5×10^6 per 10^7 cultured cells. After 4 days of in vitro incubation in the presence of absence of TRF, four culture dishes of each group were pooled and the number of antibody-producing cells was determined in triplicate with a modified Jerne plaque technique.

Assay for suppressor cell activity

Spleen cell suspension were prepared from mice that had been primed with TNP-SRBC four to six weeks earlier. Eight million cells were injected i.v. either into irradiated BALB/c-mice or to nontreated BALB/c-nude mice of different ages (6, 9 and 12 weeks old). All mice were stimulated with TNP-SRBC (1×10^8) at the same time. Ten days later the antibody-titer against TNP was determined by hemagglutination of TNP-HRBC.

RESULTS AND CONCLUSIONS

We investigated the functional maturation stage of an
enriched population of B-cells by measuring the capacity of
nude spleen cells to accept a T-cell signal in the form of
a T-cell replacing factor (TRF). By this method complicated
cell interaction is avoided since spleen cells from nude
mice of different age are stimulated in vitro by SRBC
only in the presence of TRF. In this culture method the
developmental stage of lymphocytes was defined by the time
of explantation. Since the duration of the culture is short
(4 days), further differentiation is not expected to interfere. Therefore uncontrolled helper activities of the
cellular environment is reduced in this system as compared
to irradiated hosts.

In Fig. 1 we can see the functional maturity of various
enriched B-cell populations derived from nude mice. Spleen
cells from nude mice of different ages were cultured in the
presence of antigen and TRF. TRF was obtained from adult T-
cells. After four days the magnitude of the immune response
in cultures from newborn or aged mice was compared with
cultures from 7-8 weeks old mice. It will be seen that
control cultures of nude spleen cells from adult mice yield
ten times as many PFC in the presence (B) of TRF as in its
absence (A). Unlike the control cultures without TRF, the
addition of TRF to neonatal nude spleen cells does not lead
to an increase in the number of PFC. Spleen cell - cultures
from mice, 5, 10 and 15 days old (C, D, E), do not yield
many PFC after four days. Cells which can be converted to
plasma cells in the presence of TRF seem to appear later
during ontogeny, namely in the third week (25 days) after
birth (F). We have shown that this unresponsiveness is not
caused by suppressor cells (R. Bösing-Schneider, 1979). It
is interesting to correlate this effect with the appearance
of B-cell surface markers. Since it is known that IgD molecules as well as complement- and Fc-receptors appear on
mouse spleen cells also late after birth, (Gelfand et al.,
1974; Kearney et al., 1977; Rosenberg et al., 1977), one

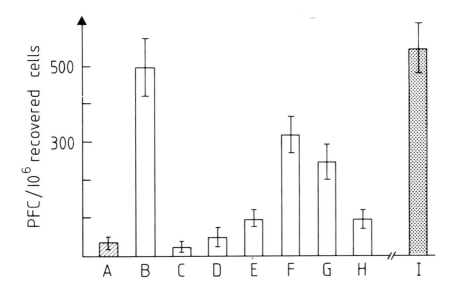

Figure 1 - AGE-RELATED CHANGES OF NUDE SPLEEN CELL FUNCTION
Spleen cells from nude mice of different ages (A,B=7 weeks;
C=5 days; D=10 days; E=15 days; F=25 days; G=12 weeks; H=16
weeks; I=control Balb/c mice, 16 weeks) were cultured in
the presence of antigen and TRF. After four days of incubation the number of plaque-forming cells was determined.

can inquire whether the receptor for the T-cell signal might
be related to them.

In order to investigate the functional state of aged
spleen cells we measured the magnitude of responsiveness in
cultures from older mice (G, H). Since under conventional
conditions the life span of nude mice is shorter than that
of normal mice, nude spleen cells were taken 12 and 16 weeks
after birth and stimulated in vitro in the presence of TRF.
If one compares the antibody response in these cultures with
the preceeding results, one can see that the capacity to produce antibodies in the presence of TRF is reduced in aged
nude spleen cells (G, H). Since spleen cells from normal
mice of this age do not show this effect (I), one can ask
whether the absence of the thymus in the nude mouse leads

120

to premature aging phenomena of nude spleen cells. Normal
animals are known to show aging effects at the age of 24
months, when the thymus epithelial cells have degenerated.
(Hirokawa and Makinodan, 1975).

It has to be investigated whether the decreased capacity of aged nude speen cells to react in vitro against sheep
red blood cells in the presence of TRF is also correlated
to the absence of surface markers or whether suppressor
cells contribute to this effect in aged nude mice. Therefore we tested in an adoptive transfer whether memory cells
of primed mice could be transferred to young and old nude
mice equally well. In Fig. 2 it is demonstrated that when
young nude mice (A) are used as hosts, transferred memory
cells can be activated as well as in irradiated hosts (D).

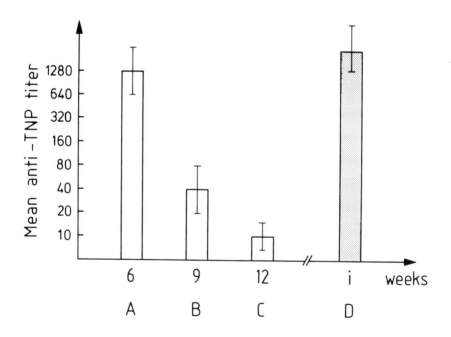

Figure 2 - EFFECT OF SUPPRESSOR CELLS IN AGED NUDE MICE ON
THE ACTIVATION OF MEMORY CELLS

Spleen cells from mice that had been primed with TNP-SRBC
were transferred either to Balb/c nude mice of different
age (A,B and C) or to irradiated syngeneic mice (D).
Ten days after antigenic challenge with TNP-SRBC the
antibody titer against TNP was determined by hemagglutination of TNP-HRBC.

This is not possible in nude mice older than 9 weeks when a decreased activity of memory cells is observed.

From this result it is concluded that suppressor cells are increased in older nude mice which might derive from a "prethymic" precursor pool, since we have shown that an increased number of PNA-positive cells can be detected in older nude mice (R. Bösing-Schneider, manuscript in preparation). Whether these cells have suppressive activity has to be studied.

REFERENCES

Bösing-Schneider, R., 1979. Functional maturation of neonatal spleen cells. Immunology 36, 527.

Click, R.E., Benck, L. and Alter, B.J. 1972. Enhancement of antibody synthesis in vitro by mercaptoethanol. Cell Immunol. 3, 156.

Gelfand, M.C., Elfenbein, G.J., Frank, M.M. and Paul, W.E., 1974. Ontogeny of B-lymphocytes. J.exp.Med. 139, 1125.

Hirokawa, K. and Makinodan, T., 1975. Thymic involution: effect on T cell differentiation. J.Immunol. 114, 1659.

Kearney, J.F., Cooper, M.D, Klein, J., Abney, E.R., Parkhouse, R.M.E. and Lawton, A.R., 1977. Ontogeny of Ia and IgD on IgM-bearing B-lymphocytes in mice. J.exp.Med. 146, 297.

Makinodan, T., 1978. Mechanism of senescence of immune responses. Fed.Proc. 37, 1239.

Rosenberg, Y.J. and Parish, C.R., 1977. Ontogeny of the antibody forming cell line in mice. IV. Appearance of cells bearing Fc-receptors, complement-receptors and surface immunoglobulin. J.Immunol. 118, 612.

Schimpl, A. and Wecker, E., 1972. Stimulation of IgG antibody response in vitro by T-cell replacing factor. J.exp. Med. 137, 547.

Segre, M. and Segre, D., 1976. Humoral Immunity in aged mice I. Age-related decline in the secondary Response to DNP of spleen cells propagated in diffusion chambers. J. Immunol. 116, 731.

Weksler, M.E., Innes, J.B. and Goldstein, G., 1978. Immunological studies of aging. IV. The contribution of thymic involution to the immune deficiencies of aging mice and reversal with thymopoietin. J.exp.Med. 148, 996.

OCCURRENCE OF NON VIABLE LYMPHOCYTES AND
IN VITRO CYTOTOXIC LYMPHOCYTES IN DYING MICE

P. Ebbesen, T. Faber and K. Fuursted

The Institute of Cancer Research
(sponsored by the Danish Cancer Society)
Radiumstationen, Nörrebrogade 44
DK-8000 Aarhus C, Denmark

SUMMARY

16-22 months old untreated CBA and C57/bl mice judged to die
within 24 hours had a higher percentage dead leukocytes in
lymph nodes, spleen and thymus than had like aged old mice
and young healthy mice. Dying CBA and DBA mice furthermore
showed enhanced in vitro cytotoxicity of spleen lymphocytes
towards syngeneic fibroblasts and YAC target cells.

INTRODUCTION

Both the events precipitating the process of dying, and the
initial bodily changes can be of very different nature.
However, irrespective of initial change there may well emerge
process common to most dying and consequently of interest for
those cases where medical intervention is desirable.

MATERIALS AND METHODS

Untreated inbred, specific pathogen free CBA, C57/bl and DBA
female mice of 2 and 16 months of age were used. All animals
were inspected 6 days a week for 6 months, and when one of the
old mice were judged to die within 24 hours that animal plus
another old but healthy looking mouse and a young mouse was
sacrificed by cervical dislocation and cells harvested immediately for dye exclusion test and cytotoxicity testing.
The latter test being carried out whenever there were 3 dying
mice on the same day.

For the supravital dye exclusion test lymphoid organs were removed and immediately placed in RPMI - 1640 with 10% heat inactivated fetal calf serum on ice. After cutting the organs with a razor blade, and shaking the suspension gently, 2 minutes were allowed for clumps to settle before 1 ml mono-cellular suspension was mixed with a similar volume of 2% nigrosin in buffered saline on ice and live and dead lympho-cytes counted. Smears, later to be Giemsa stained were also made.

Test for autoreactivity. Syngeneic embryo fibroblasts and the A strain lymphoma YAC-1 cells were used as target cells. After one wash in RPMI the pellet of 5×10^6 cells had 200 μCi ^{51}Cr and RPMI added to make a total volume of 1 ml. After 1 hour of wagging at 37°C, 5% CO_2 the cells were washed three times in phosphate buffered saline, and finally made up to 10^5/ml in RPMI. Each microtiter plate well received 1 ml of target cell suspension.

Spleen cells obtained from tumor-free spleens were washed once in RPMI and resuspended in 4 ml RPMI, and sub-sequently layered upon 3 ml Ficoll-isopaque (12 parts 14% Ficoll to 5 parts 33% isopaque), and centrifuged 15 minutes 2000 g at 20°C after the lymphocyte layer had been harvested. It was washed once in 5 ml RPMI and then resuspended in RPMI, live cells counted and made into a suspension containing 10^6 live cells per ml. This procedure removes red cells and granulocytes. One ml of the lymphocyte suspension was added to each microtiter well on top of the target cells. Lymphocytes from each mouse was added to 24 wells with labelled target cells. In addition target cells were incubated with no attack-ing cells to give spontaneous release, and labelled target cells were treated with water to give total cronium release.

The microtiter plate was kept on a wagger at 37°C, 5% CO_2 for 4 hours. Thereafter, the supernatant was harvested and counted in a gamma counter.

124

RESULTS

The mean value for the percentage of dead lymphocytes was
higher in dying than in other mice. Standard deviations were,
however, high, so the t-test indicated no difference of mean
at the 1% level. Spermans rank test indicated a difference between values for lymph nodes and spleens in CBA mice and large
thymus cells in C57/bl thymus. Most dying mice had histologic
evidence of either leukemia/reticulosarcoma or mammary tumor.
Presence or absence of malignancy did not seem to influence
the result.

Healthy old animals showed slightly higher mean value
for cellular cytotoxicity than young animals. With dying a
highly significant increase was noticed.

DISCUSSION

Although our test animals may start dying for many reasons
and must be at different time distances from spontaneous death
at the time of sacrifice, we found a general tendency for cell
suspensions made from dying animals to hold more dead lymphocytes than healthy mice of the same age. As no kinetic studies
were made we do not know if this is due to increased rate of
leukocyte dying or decreased rate of complete removal of dying
cells. Also the distribution of decay on the many functional
subpopulations of lymphocytes is unknown. An enhanced percentage of dead lymphocytes was found irrespective of the
animals showing histologic evidence of malignancy or not.
Provided that malignancy was a cause of death this suggests
that lymphocyte decay is common to death brought about by
several causes.

Our observation of enhanced autoreactivity towards
syngeneic fibroblasts and of enhanced cytotoxicity towards the
YAC-1 cells that are much in use as target for natural killer
cells suggests that self-destruction brought about by cytotoxic
lymphocytes can be part of the process of dying.

ANALYSIS OF LYMPHOID CELL DIFFERENTIATION ANTIGENS IN YOUNG AND OLD CHICKENS

G.Wick and K.Traill

Institute for General and Experimental

Pathology, University of Innsbruck, Medical

School, A - 6o2o Innsbruck, Austria

ABSTRACT

The expression of chicken lymphoid cell differentiation antigens reco gnized by turkey-anti-chicken bursa cell sera (ABS) and turkey anti-chicken thymus cell sera(ATS)was studied in indirect immunofluorescence and correlated with cell size using the FACS. The specificity of these sera in vitro has been documented by conventional techniques previously.Furthermore, ABS and ATS are able to deplete chickens of B and T cells respectively in vivo. Also on the FACS no cross reaction of ABS with T cells and ATS with B cells of normal white Leghorn (NWL) chickens was observed. In the peripheral blood of 5 week old NWL characteristic size differences emerged between B and T cells in scatter analysis, B cells being more heterogenous. Comparing 5 week and 1 year old NWL, it became obvious that (a) increasing age entails the appearance of more uniformly sized peripheral blood lymphocytes (PBL),and (b)PBL of old birds express B and T cell specific surface antigens in a significantly higher density than those of young chickens.These age-dependent changes could be mimicked in 5 week old NWL by feeding a high cholesterol diet (5kg/feed)for 1-2 weeks.At the time of this writing it is not yet established, if these cholesterol-induced alterations are reversible. Additional experiments using a fluorometer microscope rather than the FACS revealed that surface Ig is also expressed in higher density on B cells of adult (1 year) and old (3 years) as compared to young (3-12 weeks) NWL.

INTRODUCTION

This report presents first data from a project aimed at the study of possible differences in the expression of surface antigens on chicken lymphoid cells during aging. Our own interest in this species stems from work on the so called Obese strain (OS) of chickens which develop a hereditary spontaneous autoimmune thyroiditis that provides an exact model for human Hashimoto's thyroiditis (for review see Wick et al.1974,Wick et al. 1981).For these investigations allo-and xenoantisera against various surface markers of mononuclear cells were produced in this laboratory (Wick et al.,1973,Albini and Wick,1974, Albini and Wick,1975, Schauenstein and Wick,1977, Hála et al.,1979).The final goal of these studies would be the attempt to correlate possible age-dependent alterations of surface characteristics of mononuclear cells with changes in the immunologic reactivity.

towards foreign and self antigens. The degree of expression of surface antigens has – among other factors – been shown to depend on the micro-viscosity of the plasma membrane which in turn is proportionally affected by the intramembraneous ratio of free cholesterol/phospholipids (Shinitzky and Inbar,1976). It is possible that this may also be one of the factors leading to changes in lymphocyte surface determinant expression in older age (Rivnay et al.,1979).

As an initial step we have chosen to study the expression of B-cell specific and T-cell specific markers in indirect immunofluorescence (IIF) tests using anti-chicken bursa cell sera (ABS) and anti-chicken thymus cell sera (ATS). These xenoantisera were prepared in turkeys. They can not only be used for the in vitro delineation of B-and T-cells, but also for selective elimination of these subpopulations in vivo (de Carvalho et al.,1981).As an analytic tool the fluorescence activated cell sorter (FACS) was used for this part of our studies (Wick and Hála, 1981).

In a second series of experiments the expression of surface antigens reco-gnized by ABS, ATS and – in addition – anti-Ig was studied in a similar fashion, the measurements, however, being done with a fluorometer micros-cope rather than the FACS. This allows the simultaneous assessment by morphological criteria.

MATERIALS AND METHODS

Chickens:

Sex matched random bred normal White Leghorn (NWL) chickens obtained either from a local breeder or our own colony were used throughout. Their age ranged from 3 weeks to 3 years. All birds were kept under standard conditions on a 14/10 hour light/dark schedule and received the same food, except in those instances where a cholesterol-enriched diet was given.

Preparation of cells and performance of membrane IIF tests:

The preparation of bursa cells,thymocytes and PBL has been described (Albini and Wick, 1974).Membrane IIF tests were either performed in tubes for FACS analysis as described (Wick and Hála,1981) or using a semiauto-mated (Schauenstein et al.,1976) micromethod. The turkey ABS and ATS, the rabbit anti-chicken Ig serum and the FITC anti-turkey IgG and anti-rabbit IgG conjugates were the same as used in earlier work (Albini and Wick,1975) Optimal working dilutions of antisera and conjugates were determined by chessboard titrations.

Optical equipment

FACS analyses were done on a FACS II (Becton Dickinson,Sunnyvale,Ca.) using gain 4 both for scatter and fluorescence and a linear scale for display.For quantitative microfluorometry we used a Zeiss SMP 03(Zeiss,Oberkochen, FRG) interfaced with a PDP 8 microcomputer. All measurements were done on at least 250 cells per slide with a 40/0.95 dry objective.

RESULTS

Scatter and fluorescence FACS curves for PBL from a 5 week and a 1 year old male NWL are shown in figure 1.While the narrower size distribution of adult PBL is clear cut(fig.1A) the increase in fluorescence intensity of the main peaks with both ABS (fig.1B)and ATS (fig.1C) is present, albeit less pronounced. The occurrence of a dimly staining population of T cells in adult birds is a reproducible observation.
The shift in fluorescence intensity has also been substantiated by quantitative microfluorimetric analysis. As shown in figure 2 this phenomenon was not only found for antigens recognized by ABS and ATS (not shown), but also for surface Ig.
When similar experiments were performed with PBL of 5 week old NWL kept on a conventional diet or fed with a diet enriched with 1 g cholesterol/kg food a narrowing of the size distribution and a slightly increased density of determinants reacting with ABS or ATS developed in the latter group of chickens.

CONCLUSIONS

Our results have revealed characteristic age-dependent changes in size distribution and surface antigen expression on chicken B-and T-cells during aging. These changes consist in (a) a narrowing of the size distribution of PBL from adult as compared to young NWL;(b) an increase of the density of surface determinants recognized by ABS, ATS and anti-Ig.
The reasons for these alterations remain to be clarified. One conceivable underlying mechanism may be an alteration of the PBL membrane viscosity. Preliminary attempts to modulate the expression of surface antigens by a cholesterol enriched diet seem to support this hypothesis. Present experiments are aimed at substantiating these findings by in vitro modulation of the lymphocyte plasma membranes.

ACKNOWLEDGEMENTS

This work was supported by a grant from the Jubiläumsfondsprojekt der Österreichischen Nationalbank (project Nr.1613). G.Wick performed part of

128

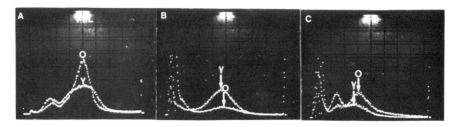

Figure 1: FACS analysis of IIF tests on suspensions of PBL of 5 week (y)
and 1 year old (o) NWL using ABS and ATS.Abscissa: Scatter and
fluorescence channels respectively. Ordinate: number of cells.

A: Scatter profiles; B: Fluorescence profiles with ABS;
C: Fluorescence profiles with ATS. For explanation see text.

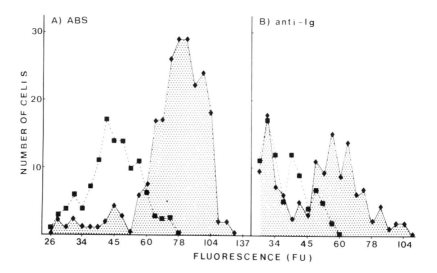

Figure 2: Histograms of microfluorimetric measurements of IIF tests on
suspensions of PBL of 7 week and 3 year (shaded) old NWL.
Panels A and B represent results of two different experiments
on the same birds. Only positively staining B cells with
fluorescence values above the background obtained with normal
sera are shown. Note shift of fluorescence intensity to higher
values in the old bird in both instances.

these slides during a visit to the Basel Institute for Immunology. The stimulating discussions with Drs.Auli and Paavo Toivanen are remembered with pleasure. We also thank Mrs.Pia Müller for her competent technical help.

REFERENCES

Schauenstein,K.,Wick, G.and Kink,H.: The micro membrane fluorescence test: a new rapid semiautomated technique based on the Microtiter[R] system. J.Immunol.Meth.10:143-150,1972.

Wick,G.and Hála,K.: Xenogeneic and allogeneic surface determinants of chicken mononuclear cells.Festschrift for N.K.Jerne (I.Lefkovits and C.Steinberg,eds.) S.Karger,Basel, 1981 (in print).

De Carvalho,L.C.,Wick,G.and Roitt,I.:Requirement of T cells for the development of spontaneous autoimmune thyroiditis in Obese strain (OS) chickens.J.Immunol. (in print)

Albini,B.and Wick,G.:Delineation of T and B lymphoid cells in the chicken. J.Immunol.112:444-450 (1974).

Albini,B.and Wick,G.: Ontogeny of lymphoid cell surface determinants in the chicken.Int.Arch.Allergy 48:513-529 (1975).

Hála,K.,Vilhelmová,M.,Schumannová,J.and Plachý,J.:A new recombinant allele in the B complex of the chicken.Fol.Biol.(Praha)25:323-324(1979).

Rivnay,B.,Globerson,A.and Shinitzky,M.:Viscosity of lymphocyte plasma membrane in aging mice and its possible relation to serum cholesterol Mech.Aging Develop.10:71-79 (1979)

Schauenstein,K.and Wick,G.:Surface antigens of chicken white blood cells detected by heterologous antisera; In SOLOMON and HORTON eds.,Developmental Immunobiology,pp363-369 (Elsevier/North Holland,Biomedical Press,Amsterdam,1977).

Shinitzky,M.and Inbar,M.:Microviscosity parameters and protein mobility in biological membranes.Bochim.Biophys.Acta 433:133-149 (1976).

Wick,G.,Albini,B.and Milgrom,F.:Antigeneic surface determinants of chicken lymphoid cells.I.Serologic properties of anti-bursa and anti-thymus sera.Clin.Exp.Immunol.15:237-250 (1973)

Wick,G.,Sundick,R.S.and Albini,B.:The Obese strain (OS)of chickens: An animal model with spontaneous autoimmune thyroiditis.Clin.Immunol. Immunopathol.3:272-300 (1974).

Wick,G.,Albini,B.and Johnson,W.:Antigenic surface determinants of chicken lymphoid cells.II.Selective in vivo and in vitro activity of anti-bursa and anti-thymus sera.Immunol.28:305-313 (1975)

Wick,G.,Boyd,R.,Hála,K.,Pontes de Carvalho,L.C.,Kofler,R.,Müller,P.-U.and Cole,R.K.: The Obese strain (OS) of chickens with spontaneous autoimmune thyroiditis.Review of recent data.Current Topics Microbiol. and Immunol.(in print).

AGE DEPENDENCE OF T LYMPHOCYTES IN ALTAMURANA'S SHEEP[1]

R.Celi,E.Jirillo,A.De Santis,G.Martemucci and P.Montemurro

Istituto di Zootecnia-Facolta' di Agraria-and

Istituto di Microbiologia-Facoltà di Medicina-

Università di Bari,70100,Italy

ABSTRACT

The frequency of E-rosette cells(T lymphocytes from peripheral blood)has been evaluated in ewes,as function of ageing.Results have shown a significant decrease of E-rosettes in aged animals(up to 9 years old),which paral= lels the decrement of the total number of peripheral lympho= cytes.Furthermore,studies on the same group of animals indicate that in lactating ewes the percentage of E-ros= ettes is a little higher,even if not significant,than that from dry ewes.

INTRODUCTION

Nowadays,many systems,manifesting age related depen= dence,are being investigated in order to augment our knowledge of the effects of ageing at the cellular and molecular levels.One of these is the immune system,whose normal activities decline with age and the decline appe= ars to be a characteristic of the more evoluted animals.

[1] The present work was supported by the Italian National Research Council:contract n.79.00213.80(Progetto fina= lizzato"Difesa delle risorse genetiche delle popolazio= ni animali;"Sub-progetto"Interazione genotipo-ambiente nel quadro delle attitudini produttive e riproduttive degli ovini".

In this respect,the observations made in humans and ani=
mals are numerous and conflicting(Makinodan,1980;Makinodan and Kay,
1980).What is clear is that the onset and the rate of decline vary
with the type of immune function and the species and,parallelly to
the decreased performance of the immune system,the incidence of in=
fectious diseases,autoimmune and immune-complex diseases and cancer
increases(Makinodan,1980).
In the present work the frequency of T lymphocytes,using the E-roset=
ting method,and the absolute number of lymphocytes in the peripheral
blood of lactating and dry ewes will be studied,as function of ageing.

MATERIALS AND METHODS

   Animals:altamurana's ewes,lactating and dry,have been employed
and grouped as follows:

Years	1	2	3	4	5	6	7	8	9	Total number
n° of lactating ewes	-	-	4	5	-	-	6	2	8	25
n° of dry ewes	18	13	-	6	9	-	6	2	7	61

Lymphocyte separation:blood samples were taken from the jugular vein
and heparinized.Blood was diluted 5 times with Hank's Balanced Salt
Solution(HBSS) and layered in a gradient of Ficoll/Hypaque according
to Böyum(1968).After centrifuging at 200xg for 30 min the lymphocyte
layer was removed and washed 3 times in HBSS.
Rosette test:it was carried out according to Binns(1978).Briefly,
$2x10^6$ lymphocytes were added to 20 μl of 2% homologous Sheep Red
Blood Cells(SRBC) in the enhancing medium(4% Dextran 150),mixed vi=
gorously,centrifuged at 200xg for 5 min and incubated overnight at 4
°C.Rosettes were defined as bearing 4 or more adherent SRBC.A stan=
dard donor was employed in each experiment.

In another set of experiments E-rosettes were determined using either autologous or homologous SRBC. The total number of peripheral leuko= cytes/mm^3 was counted in a Bürker chamber.Differential counts were performed on peripheral blood fimls stained with Giemsa.

RESULTS

Table 1 illustrates the age related decrement of E-rosettes in 86 ewes.The percentage of E-rosettes was maximal in animals 1 and 2 years old(all dry) and gradually decreased in more aged individuals(up to 9 years old).In lactating animals(7,8,9 years old) the percentage of E-rosettes was a little higher,even if not statistically signifi= cant,than that of the respective dry ewes.

TABLE 1-TOTAL NUMBER OF LYMPHOCYTES AND PERCENTAGE OF E-ROSETTES IN
LACTATING AND DRY EWES(Means ± S.D.)

Age (years)	Lymphocytes/mm^3		%RFC*	
	Lactating	Dry	Lactating	Dry
1		9248 ± 3064		17 ± 7
2		7059 ± 1317		13 ± 4
3	7574 ± 162	6808 ± 1653	9 ± 6	
4	5426 ± 517	5228 ± 2880	5 ± 1	8 ± 4
5		5547 ± 2393		6 ± 3
7	4250 ± 951	4857 ± 591	4 ± 3	2 ± 2
8	4000 ± 893	5170 ± 1660	4 ± 5	1 ± 1
9	5187 ± 1912	4684 ± 1420	5 ± 3	2 ± 2

* RFC= Rosette-Forming Cells

It is worth to mention that in the earlier periods of life(1-2 years) the percentage of rosetting cells had a very broad range,likely due to some lymphocyte populations with a still low affinity for SRBC,while in the following ages values are more closed each other.Table 1 also shows that the total number of peripheral blood lymphocytes/mm^3 de= creased,as function of ageing.Furthermore,the parallel decrement of E-rosettes and lymphocytes also emerges from the coefficient of cor= relation(r=0.63 for lactating ewes and r=0.50 for dry ewes),which is significant for P<0.0 1.

Table 2 shows the percentage of E-rosette cells obtained using auto= logous and homologous SRBC.The number of rosettes was quite similar in both cases,in the sense that values were a little lower in the presence of homologous SRBC.This fact may indicate that no allo-anti= genic determinants are involved in the interaction lymphocyte/SRBC.

TABLE 2- E-ROSETTE FORMATION BY OVINE LYMPHOCYTES WITH AUTOLOGOUS AND HOMOLOGOUS SRBC.

| Sheep no. | % RFC | |
	Autologous SRBC	Homologous SRBC
1	12	9
2	15	12
3	18	15
4	19	17

CONCLUSIONS

Until now,few studies have been carried out on E-rosette formati= on with peripheral blood lymphocytes of sheep.The major difficulty encountered has been represented by the failure of these cells to bind erythrocytes from any species.However,just recently Binns(1978) has developed a method based on the use of dextran wich enhances the binding between SRBC and homologous ovine lymphocytes.The available data confirm the thymus dependence of the rosetting lymphocytes.

In the present study we have taken advantage of the aforementioned procedure in order to determine the percentage of E-rosettes and the total number of circulating lymphocytes of altamurana's sheep at different ages.Our data yielded a significant decrease of E-ro= settes with age and parallelly a low number of lymphocytes in older animals.Now,the interpretation of these findings is under way.We can postulate that a progressive loss of T cell subsets occurs with age,which leads to the decrement of E-rosettes.On the other hand, aside from the reduced number of circulating lymphocytes,we cannot exclude that also the affinity of lymphocytes for SRBC might dimi= nish with age.

In contrast with our data Binns has found an increase of E-rosettes in sheep,as function of ageing.Such a discrepancy may depend on two points:1) dietary factors which may affect the immune system (Maki= nodan and Kay,1980;Wick,1980);2) use of breeds with different gene= tical features when compared to our breed.In this respect,we have previous experience of the influence of different ovine genotypes on some functional parameters of blood cells as well as the SRBC electrophoretic mobility(Celi et al.,1978).

It is very interesting that our results are in good accordance with Alexopoulos and Babitis(1976),Kishimoto et al.,(1978),and Burghart-Czaplinska et al.,(1980) data about the age dependence of T lympho= cytes in humans.Therefore,we believe that sheep may represent a sui= table animal model for studying the mechanisms of ageing of the im= mune system together with other physiological parameters,even inclu= ding the zootechnical ones(milk,meat,wool et cetera production).

AKNOWLEDGEMENTS

We are grateful to Mr. Angelo Navarra for his skilful technical assistance.

REFERENCES

Alexopoulos,C.and Babitis,P.:Age dependence of T lym-
    phocytes.Lancet 1:426,1976
Binns,R.M.:Sheep erythrocytes rosettes in pigs,sheep ,
    cattles and goats demonstrated in the presence of
    dextran.J.Immunol. Method.21:197-210,1978
Böyum,A.:Separation of leukocytes from blood and bone
    marrow with specifical reference to factors which
    influence and modify sedimentation properties of
    hematopoietic cells.Scand.J.Clin.Lab.Invest. 21:
    Suppl.97,9-109,1968
Burghart-Czaplinska,M.,Sawicka,B.,Lewandowska,J.,and
    Danowska,A.:Immunobiology of ageing.I.Some immu=
    nological changes in aged persons.4th Internatio=
    nal Congress of Immunology-Paris,Abstracts,1980
Celi,R.,Jirillo,E.,and Schiavone M.:La mobilita' elet=
    troforetica degli eritrociti ovini.Prime ricerche
    per la sua caratterizzazione in relazione ad ipo=
    tesi applicative nel campo zootecnico.Zoot.Nutr.
    Anim.4:47-53,1978
Kishimoto,S.,Tomino,S.,Inomata,K.,Kotegawa,S.,Saito,T.,
    Kuroki,M.,Mitsuya,H.,and Hisamitsu,S.:Age-related
    changes in the subsets and functions of human T
    lymphocytes.J.Immunol.121:1773-1780,1978
Makinodan,T.:Immunodeficiencies and ageing.In:The im=
    mune system:Functions and therapy of dysfunctions.
    Ed.G.Doria,and A.Eskol,pp.55-63(Academic Press,
    1980)
Makinodan,T.,and Kay M.M.B.:Age influence on the immune
    system.Advan.Immunol. 29:257-330;1980
Wick,G.:Analysis of chicken lymphoid cell differentia=
    tion antigens with the fluorescence activated cell
    sorter(FACS).Communication presented at the"Inter=
    national workshop on Immunology and Ageing-Ancona,
    September,1980

SESSION IV

THYMIC ENDOCRINE ACTIVITY AND AGEING.

THYMIC HORMONES AND AGING

Mireille Dardenne, Marie-Anne Bach and Jean-François Bach

INSERM U 25 - Hôpital Necker

161, rue de Sèvres - 75015 Paris - France

ABSTRACT

The level of the serum thymic factor (FTS) measured by the rosette inhibition assay, and of other circulating thymic hormones, declines with advancing age both in mice and in man. This decline is accelerated in auto-immune prone mice. These data are quite consistant with the intrinsic deficiency of thymic secretory activity present with aging. It is corroborated by the decrease of specific binding of anti-FTS antibodies to thymic reticulo-epithelial cells, as detected by indirect immunofluorescence. One shoud note that, in addition to the decline in thymic hormone secretion, environmental factors, such as serum inhibitors, probably play a significant role in the age-associated disappearance of FTS. In any case, it is highly plausible that the disappearance of thymic hormones is one of the major causes for T cell impairment observed in aged animals or humans. Further studies will attempt to establish if lifelong administration of thymic hormones prevents senescence of the immune system.

INTRODUCTION

The major role of the thymus in the development of the immune system was revealed through the study of the effects of neonatal thymectomy in experimental animals performed by Miller (1961), Good et al. (1962) and Jankovic (1962). The consequences of neonatal and adult thymectomy and the resulting physiological and biochemical alterations and deficiencies have then been ultimately studied by many investigators and have permitted to establish that the thymus has an endocrine role. However, Osoba and Miller (1963) were the first to present convicing evidence that a humoral thymic factor is responsible for T cell maturation when they showed that the impaired immune system of neonatally thymectomized mice can be restored by implanting intraperitoneally cell-impermeable Millipore diffusion chambers containing a thymic tissue. Subsequently, more refined studies demonstrated that the thymus secretes hormone-like substances that can transform precursor cells into T cells and drive immature T cells further along in their differentiation. Recently, a number of laboratories presented convincing data demonstrating the stimulation of immunocompetence of thymectomized mice by injection of thymic extracts (Bach and Carnaud, 1976 ; Bach, 1979)

Major progress has now been achieved concerning both the chemical nature
and the biological significance of thymic factors. It has permitted to en-
visage the therapeutical applications of these factors (or hormones) in
various clinical conditions associated with T cell deficiencies.

AGE-DEPENDENCY OF SERUM THYMIC FACTOR LEVEL

The thymus involution begins around the time of sexual maturity in
humans and in mice (Good and Gabrielson, 1964). Not long thereafter, some
immunological activities begin to decline (Makinodan et al., 1971) and an
increase in the incidence of autoimmunity, infections and cancer is observed. The immunodeficiency observed in aging seems to be due primarily (but
not solely) to changes in T cell sub-populations (Adler et al., 1971 ;
Konen et al., 1973 ; Kishmoto, 1969). In fact, some of these age-related
defects in immune functions can be reversed by a thymus gland, thymocytes from young donors or by thymic hormones.

Parallel to this decline in the thymic mass and this alteration in T
cell functions, thymic hormone level progressively diminishes.

Presence of thymic hormones in peripheral blood

Thymic hormones are produced by the thymic epithelium (this has now
been directly demonstrated by immunofluorescence using antisera directed
at thymosin α1 (Hirokawa and Saitoh, 1981) and facteur thymique sérique
(FTS)(Monier et al., 1980). One may detect humoral activity in peripheral
blood and assays have been set up which allow to evaluate the serum level
of thymic hormones. In fact, it is from serum that FTS was initially isolated (before being chemically isolated and characterized from thymic extracts, with identical amino acid composition). Recently, in a more indirect fashion, evidence has been brought that thymopoietin and thymosin α1
also circulate in the blood. The significance of the thymic hormone-like
activity of circulating prealbumin (Burton et al., 1978)is not yet well
understood. It is probable but not definitively known if it is explained by the transport of a small thymic peptide such as FTS, as we have
recently suggested on several experimental arguments (Dardenne et al.,1980)

Evaluation of blood levels

Several methods have been described to measure the levels of circulating thymic hormones. The first of these methods was described in our laboratory in 1972 (Bach and Dardenne, 1972a).It is based on the changes induced by thymic hormones on the minority of spleen cells of adult thymectomized mice which form spontaneous rosettes with sheep erythrocytes. The

assay consists in detecting the smallest serum concentration which renders
spleen rosette-forming cells (RFC) sensitive to antitheta serum (AθS) or to
azathioprine, the well-known immunosuppressive agent that happens to inhibit, at low concentration, rosette formation in normal mice and to lose
this property, as AθS does,in adult thymectomized (ATx) mice (Bach and Dardenne, 1972b).Results are expressed in serum dilutions ; the higher the
active dilution, the higher the concentration of the hormone. Sera are used
in the tests after ultrafiltration on Amicon membranes (mol wt cut-off
50,000) to remove high mol wt inhibitors. In selected cases, the relationship of the activity detected to FTS may be verified by passing the serum
on an immunoadsorbant prepared with an antibody raised against synthetic
FTS. The strict thymus dependency of the activity detected by the rosette
assay is demonstrated by its total absence in the serum of nude or thymectomized (Tx) mice and of patients with Di George syndrome, and its reappearance in all individuals after thymus grafting.

A similar method has been described in 1977 by Twomey et al. Serum is
incubated with nude mouse spleen cells and the increase in θ-positive cells
is measured using a cytotoxic assay with Trypan blue. The sensitivity of
the test is increased by adding ubiquitin at subliminal concentration, a
protein known to induce non-specifically T (and B) cell markers. Serum ul-
trafiltrates are used, as in the rosette assay, rather than total serum,
because of the presence of serum inhibitors. Thymopoietin shows activity in
the test. Interestingly, FTS whose effects are inhibited by ubiquitin
(Iwata et al.,1979) is not active in the test. Results are expressed in ng-
equivalent of thymopoietin, which does not take full account of other molecules than thymopoietin which could be active in the test, and of the inter-
fering molecules (carrier proteins, inhibitors...). As for the rosette
assay, the specificity of the Twomey assay is assessed by its negativity in
the sera of nude and Tx mice, and sera from patients with Di George syndrome.

Radioimmunoassays (RIA) have been described for three well-defined
thymic peptides : α 1 thymosin (Goldstein, unpublished results), FTS (Pléau
et al., 1978) and thymopoietin (Goldstein, 1976). Such RIA have not yet
been successfully applied to the evaluation of serum samples for FTS and
thymopoietin, essentially due to unsolved interference with serum proteins.
More conclusive results have been reported for α1 thymosin (Mc Clure et al.
1980), but one still awaits unequivocal demonstration of total absence of
RIA-positive material in the serum of Tx animals or humans, compared to

normal individuals, as has been obtained for the two bioassays mentioned
above.

Influence of aging on blood levels

In the mouse, the age-dependency of FTS serum level has been extensively studied. FTS is already present at adult's level at birth. Studies in
Tx pregnant mothers have shown that FTS is first detectable at the 14th day
of pregnancy. The serum level of FTS shows a discontinuous evolution with
age with three phases : a plateau level from birth until the age of 4-5
months, a sharp decline between 4 and 7 months, and finally a long terminal
phase without any detectable circulating FTS, even after concentration of
the serum (Fig.1). Similar results have been confirmed with the rosette
assay by other investigators (Iwata et al., 1979). This age-dependent
decline parallels that of thymus weight.

In man, the age-dependency of FTS level is also observed with a stable
level until the age of 15-20 years, followed by a progressive decline. The
data that we initially reported for FTS in 1972 (Bach et al., 1972) has
been confirmed with the rosette assay by other groups (Garaci et al., 1978;
Lewis et al., 1978) as well as with the Twomey assay (Twomey et al.,1977)
with similar kinetics. At variance with these data the level of thymosin α1
seems to drop earlier than that of FTS, with a decline starting as soon as
10 years of age (Goldstein et al., unpublished results).

Mechanism of FTS disappearance with aging

The presence of thymic hormones in the circulation has probably a physiological significance since adult thymectomy-induced changes may take
place as early as 5 days after thymectomy (Bach et al.,1971a) and are completely corrected in vitro by addition of thymic hormones (Bach et al.,1971b)
One may hypothesize that T cells which leave the thymus are not yet completely mature and still depend partly on circulating thymic hormones to ter-
minate their maturation. Similarly, the disappearance of FTS with aging
could represent a major factor in the T cell impairment observed in aged
animals (Bach & Beaurain,1977;Walford,1974;Kay et al., 1976).

It should be emphasized, however, that there exists an interesting and
unexplained difference in the relationship between the serum level of FTS
and azathioprine sensitivity of lymph nodes and spleen RFC of ATx and aging
mice. There is in ATx mice a rapid drop in spleen RFC sensitivity to azathioprine or AθS, as soon as the 6th day after thymectomy, parallel to the
disappearance of serum FTS. Conversely, in aging mice, the absence of FTS

does not correlate with changes in azathioprine or AθS sensitivity of spleen or lymph nodes (Bach et al., 1973). One may explain this difference by assuming that FTS controls spleen RFC-azathioprine sensitivity, but that a very low level is necessary for normal or subnormal azathioprine or AθS sensitivity of spleen RFC. Such a threshold is perhaps lower than the lowest serum levels detected by our technique. Aging mice could have a normal aza-thioprine spleen RFC sensitivity in spite of a very low (undetectable) FTS level. Another possibility relates to the presence of serum inhibitors of FTS which would mask FTS presence in the serum of aging mice.

Serum inhibitors and aging

Several observations argue in favor of the existence in normal serum of FTS inhibitors that are detectable in the rosette assay but could also alter the physiological effects of circulating thymic hormones. Total mouse serum examined in the rosette assay described above does not possess the activity reported for serum ultrafiltrate. This activity only appears after elimination of molecules with mol wt between 100,000 and 300,000 by use of diafiltration on Amicon membranes (Bach et al., 1978). These data suggest that there exists in the serum a FTS inhibitor with high mol wt which is separable from FTS by simple dialysis or diafiltration. The molecule respon-sible for this inhibitory activity of normal serum has not yet been charac-terized. It is active at very low concentrations since total serum diluted 1/5000 keeps its inhibitory activity.

Other FTS inhibitors of lower mol wt have been demonstrated when ultra-filtered serum is concentrated and chromatographed on G-25 Sephadex : the total activity of separated fractions is increased in relation to the ini-tial sample, indicating the presence of low mol wt (ultrafiltrable) inhibi-tors. In fact, using an inhibitor assay identical to that described above, we have shown the existence of two inhibitors with approximate mol wt of 4,000 and 20,000 respectively.

The largest inhibitor is removed before evaluating the serum thymic level, but the smallest ones are not eliminated and interfere with the final biological evaluation of serum FTS level. The level of high mol wt inhibi-tor has been found similar in young and old mice, but the activity of lower mol wt inhibitors has not yet been evaluated in aging mice. Their possible role in the disappearance of FTS and the paradoxical persistance of azathio-prine-RFC sensitivity has not yet been investigated.

In fact, recent studies have shown that, in addition to an intrinsic deficiency of thymic secretion, serum factors probably play a role in the disappearance of circulating FTS with age (Bach and Beaurain, 1979). When comparing the serum FTS level in mice of different ages and different strains and the ability of syngeneic thymus grafts to restore the serum FTS level in young ATx recipients, it was observed that such ability decreased progressively after birth but did not disappear completely in old mice, at least not until the age of 15 months, although at this age no more circulating factor could be detected in the serum of thymus graft donors. These data, which are reminiscent of those of Hirokawa and Makinodan (1975) suggest the existence of an external influence on the age-associated disappearance of FTS. This hypothesis has been confirmed by further experiments demonstrating that the serum FTS level obtained when a newborn thymus is grafted into young ATx recipients is higher than that reached in old normal recipients receiving a similar newborn thymus graft. The inhibitory effect of the aging mouse environment may be explained by two hypotheses : 1/ the thymus secretion is influenced by age-associated hormonal changes, in keeping with the well documented relationship between endocrine glands and the development of the immune system (Fabris, 1977) 2/ the biological activity of FTS is inhibited by factors present in old mouse serum, but not in young mouse serum, whatever the mechanism of this inhibition (enzymatic degradation, binding to a carrier protein, inhibiting factors acting at the level of the target cell).

DIRECT DEMONSTRATION OF THE DECLINE IN FTS PRODUCTION BY THYMIC EPITHELIUM WITH AGING

We have recently directly shown the presence of FTS in the thymic epithelium by use of anti-FTS antibody produced against the synthetic FTS coupled to bovine serum albumin (BSA) (Pléau et al., 1977). This antiserum was purified by the use of a FTS gel immunoabsorbent in order to remove anti-BSA antibodies. The purified antibodies were shown, by indirect immunofluorescence, to localize on the mouse thymic epithelium, and more precisely on reticulo-epithelial thymic cells (Monier et al., 1980). The specificity of the anti-FTS antibody binding was assessed by its inhibition by synthetic FTS and by the absence of binding to cultures of fibroblasts or other cells.

The binding of anti-FTS antibodies to reticulo-epithelial cells is clearly reduced in aging mice, both for the number of fluorescent cells,

and the intensity of fluorescence (Dardenne et al., 1980). These data show
that the age-dependent decline of FTS production by the thymic epithelium
parallels the FTS disappearance with aging.

PREMATURE AGE-DEPENDENT LOSS OF FTS IN PATHOLOGIC MICE

Autoimmune mice : NZB and B/W (F_1) mice have a normal level of FTS at
birth but FTS level decreases prematurely between the 3rd and 6th week of
life (Bach et al., 1973). At two months of age, NZB and B/W mice have no
significant circulating FTS. Six weeks after the decline of FTS, NZB mice
show disappearance of θ-positive lymph node RFC and a progressive decrease
in their spleen RFC sensitivity to AθS and azathioprine. This change in
spleen RFC properties is more important than in aging mice. Interestingly,
the normal sensitivity of spleen and lymph node RFC is reconstituted by
in vitro and in vivo treatment by thymic extracts.

Similarly, Swan mice, a mouse strain genetically selected from outbred
mice for its predisposition to develop antinuclear factors, also shows an
early disappearance of circulating FTS, as compared to the original Swiss
mouse population from which it is derived (Dardenne et al., 1977). Serum
levels of FTS have been studied in two other autoimmune strains of mice :
MRL/1 and MRL/Mp (Zinkernagel, 1977). FTS serum levels are much lower in
young MRL mice than in non autoimmune strains. The MRL/1 strain develops
the most severe disease and also shows the earliest FTS decline. (Unpublished results)

Hypopituitary dwarf mice : Hypopituitary dwarf mice have an hypotropic
thymus, a decreased number of circulating lymphocytes and a lymphocytic
depletion of the thymus-dependent areas of their peripheral lymphoid organs
(Fabris et al.,1972). Pelletier et al.,(1976) have found that these mice
lack FTS at an early age. These data would suggest that thymic function is
under hormonal control. Treatment of dwarf mice (Fabris et al.,1972) with
growth hormone during the first 30 days after weaning significantly prolongs
their life span, provided the thymus is not removed before the hormonal
treatment is applied. Taken together, these results suggest that the action
of some hormones on dwarf mice, such as a growth hormone and possibly thyroxine, is mediated by the release of thymic hormones which could therefore
be considered as potential contributors to the general endocrinological
homeostasis.

CORRECTION OF THE AGE-ASSOCIATED DEFICIT OF THYMIC HORMONE PRODUCTION.
Cell grafting
Grafting a thymus in a young Tx animal corrects the effect of adult
thymectomy both for serum FTS levels and spleen RFC senstivity to azathioprine and AθS. Normalization of RFC sensitivity to azathioprine occurs
simultaneously with reappearance of serum FTS on day 3 post-grafting and
reaches its maximum on day 4 (1/64 - 1/28) (Bach et al.,1973). Multiple
thymus grafts are associated with increased FTS level, grossly proportional
to the number of thymic lobes grafted, which confirms the absence of thymic
hormone-induced feed-back regulation of the thymus, already suspected from
macroscopic studies of the thymus (Tubiana et al.,1979). One should note,
however, as previously discussed, that newborn thymus grafted in old mice
is less efficient in restoring serum FTS levels than in young Tx recipients (Bach and Beaurain, 1979).

Chemotherapy
Only few immuno-restorative agents have been tested in aging animals.
There has been yet no systematic study of the effect of thymic hormones on
immunologic aging. Nevertheless, the potentials of positively influencing
thymic function by giving either thymic hormone or agents increasing its
production are enormous. Growth hormone has recently been found to result
in a several fold increase in serum levels of thymosin α 1 given to growth
hormone-deficient patients (Wara, personnal communication). Similar results
were obtained by Fabris et al. (1980) who showed that the low levels of FTS
observed in hypopituitary immunodeficient young mice were corrected by treatment with growth hormone, and thyroxine, while the undetectable FTS
levels recorded in presenescent mice were reconstituted to young values by
2-3 daily injection of L-thyroxine. Note, lastly, that FTS production provided by transplanting a presenescent thymus in ATx mice is much faster and
higher if the thymus donor has been pretreated with L-thyroxine.

This result suggests that certain hormones could correct the immunological deficit associated with aging by a direct interaction with the endocrine function of the thymus. More recent experiments have shown that a
stimulation of thymic humoral function could also be obtained by non hormonal products such as cyclomunine, a cyclic immunomodulating peptide
(Dardenne et al., 1980)/ A single injection of cyclomunine induces in normal young mice a rapid and progressive increase in FTS level. The earliest
significant rise is noted 14 days after injection and the maximum level

(more than 100 times the normal value) observed from days 90 to 150. The same FTS increase is observed in aging mice and NZB mice with similar kinetics. The thymic dependence of FTS variation is assessed by the prevention of cyclomunine induced variations in FTS levels by thymectomy. We have also shown, using indirect immunofluorescence, that the number of cells binding the antibody directed at synthetic FTS is increased by cyclomunin treatment in aging mice. Studies in progress will attempt to establish the consequences of this thymic stimulation on immunologic aging.

CONCLUSION

The level of circulating thymic hormones, such as FTS, declines in aging individuals and mice. This disappearance could be an important factor in the T cell impairment observed in aged animals. Several age-associated immune defects could be improved or reversed by administration of thymic factors. Future studies are necessary to determine whether lifelong maintenance of the serum thymic hormone levels found during early life, by repeated and lifelong administration of thymic hormones, will prevent the senescence of the immune response.

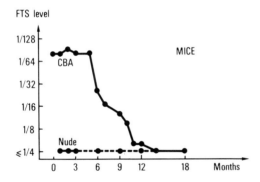

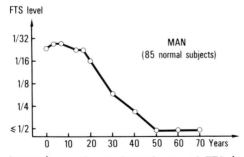

Figure 1 - Comparison of age dependency of FTS in mice and in man

REFERENCES

Adler,W.H.,Takiguchi,T. and Smith,T.T. 1971. Effect of age upon primary alloantigen recognition by mouse spleen. J.Immunol.,107: 1357-1362.

Bach,J.F., 1979. Thymic hormones. J.Immunopharmacol., 1(3) : 277-310.

Bach,J.F., Dardenne, M. and Davies,A.J.S. 1971a.Early effect of adult thymectomy. Nature, New Biology, 231 : 110-111.

Bach,J.F., Dardenne,M., Goldstein,A.L. and White,A. 1971b. Appearance of T cell markers in bone marrow rosette forming cells after incubation with purified thymosin, a thymic hormone. Proc.Natl.Acad.Sci.,U.S.A. 68 : 2734-2738.

Bach,J.F. and Dardenne,M. 1972a. Thymus dependency of rosette forming cells Evidence of a circulating thymic hormone. Transpl.Proc. 4: 345-350.

Bach,J.F. and Dardenne,M. 1972b. Antigen recognition by T lymphocytes. II. Similar effects of azathioprine, ALS and AθS on rosette forming lymphocytes in normal and neonatally thymectomized mice. Cell.Immunol. 3 : 11-21.

Bach,J.F., Dardenne, M., Papiernik,M., Barois,A., Levasseur,P. and Le Brigand,H. 1972. Evidence for a serum factor produced by the human thymus. Lancet, 2 : 1056-1058.

Bach,J.F. and Dardenne,M. 1973. Studies on thymus products. II. Demonstration and characterization of a circulating thymic hormone. Immunology, 25: 353-366.

Bach,J.F., Dardenne,M. and Salomon,J.C. 1973. Studies on thymus products. IV. Absence of serum "thymic activity" in adult NZB and (NZBxNZW)F$_1$ mice. Clin.Exp.Immunol., 14 : 247-256.

Bach,J.F. and Carnaud,C. 1976. Thymic factors. Progress in Allergy, 21 : 342-408.

Bach,J.F., Bach,M.A., Blanot,D., Bricas,E., Charreire,J., Dardenne, M., Fournier,C. and Pléau,J.M. 1978. Thymic serum factor (FTS). Bull.Inst. Pasteur, 76 : 325-398.

Bach,M.A. and Beaurain,G. 1979.Respective influence of extrinsic and intrinsic factors on the age-related decrease of thymic secretion. J.Immunol., 122 : 2505-2507.

Burton,P., Iden,S., Mitchell,K. and White,A. 1978. Thymic hormone-like restoration by human prealbumin or azathioprine sensitivity of spleen cells from thymectomized mice. Proc.Natl.Acad.Sci.USA, 75 : 823-826.

Dardenne,M., Monier,C., Biozzi,G. and Bach,J.F. 1974. Studies on thymus products. V. Influence of genetic selection based on antibody production on thymus hormone production. Clin.Exp.Immunol.,17: 339-344.

Dardenne,M., Pléau,J.M.and Bach,J.F. 1980a. Evidence of the presence in normal serum of a carrier of the serum thymic factor (FTS). Eur.J. Immunol. 10 : 83-86.

Dardenne, M., Niaudet,P., Simon-Lavoine,N. and Bach,J.F. 1980b. Stimulation of thymic humoral function by cyclomunine, a cyclic peptide, in mice. Int.J.Immunopharmacol.,2: 154-157.

Fabris,N., Pierpaoli,W. and Sorkin,E. 1972. Lymphocytes, hormones and aging Nature, 240 :557-559.

Fabris,N. 1977. Hormones and aging. in "Comprehensive Immunology".I.Immunology and Aging. T.Makinodan and E.Yunis,eds. Plenum Press, New York, pp. 73-89.

Fabris,N. and Mac Chegiani,E. 1980. Homeostatic control of thymic factor turn-over. 4th Intern.Congress of Immunology, Paris, Abstr.3-3-08.

Garaci,E., Ronchetti,R.,Del Gobbio,V.,Tramutoli,G.,Rinaldi-Garaci,C. and Imperato,C. 1978. Decreased serum thymic factor activity in asthmatic children. J.Allergy Clin.Immunol. 62 : 357-362.

Goldstein,G. 1976. Radioimmunoassay for thymopoietin. J.Immunol.117:690-692

Good,R.A., Dalmasso,A.P., Martinez,C., Archer,O.K., Pierce,J.C. and Papermaster,B.W. 1962. The role of the thymus in development of immunologic capacity in rabbits and mice. J.Exp.Med. 116: 773-796.

Good,R.A. and Gabrielson,A.B. 1964. Thymus in Immunobiology. Hoeber-Harper, New York.

Hirokawa,K. and Makinodan,T. 1975. Thymic involution. Effect of T cell differentiation. J.Immunol. 114: 1650-1655.

Hirokawa,K. and Saitoh,I. 1980. Heterogeneity of thymic epithelial cells, revealed by localization of thymosin α1 and various hydrolytic enzymes in human thymus. 4th Intern. Congress of Immunology, Paris, Abstr. 3-3-14.

Iwata,T., Incefy,G.S. and Good,R.A. 1979a. Interaction between thymopoietin and facteur thymique sérique in the rosette inhibition assay. Biochem. Biophys. Res.Com., 88 : 1419-1427.

Iwata,T., Incefy,G.S., Tanaka,T., Fernandes,G., Menendez-Botet,C.J. and Good,R.A. 1979b. Circulating thymic hormone levels in zinc deficiency. Cell.Immunol. 47 : 100-105.

Jankovic,B.D., Waksman,B.H. and Arnason,B.G. 1962. Role of the thymus in immune reactions in rats. I. The immunologic response of bovine serum albumin (antibody formation, Arthus reactivity, and delayed hypersensitivity) in rats thymectomized or splenectomized at various times after birth. J.Exp.Med. 116: 159-176.

Kay,M.B. and Makinodan,T. 1976. Immunobiology of aging. Evaluation of current status. Clin.Immunol.Immunopathol. 6: 394-397.

Kishimoto,S., Tsuyuguchi,I. and Yamamura,I. 1969. Immune response in aged mice. Clin.Exp.Immunol., 5: 525-530.

Konen,T.G., Smith,G.S. and Walford,R.L. 1973. Decline in mixed lymphocyte reactivity of spleen cells from aged mice of a long-lived strain. J.Immunol., 110: 1216-1221.

Lewis,V.M., Twomey,J.J., Bealmear,P.N., Goldstein,G. and Good,R.A. 1978. Age, thymic involution and circulating thymic hormone activity. J.Clin.Endocr. Metabol., 47: 145-150.

Makinodan,T., Perkins,E.H. and Chen,M.G. 1971. Immunologic activity of the aged. Adv.Gerontol.Res. 3: 171-198.

Mc Clure,J.E. and Goldstein,A.L. 1980. Changes with age in blood levels of thymosin α1 as measured by radioimmunoassay. 4th Intern.Gongress of Immunology, Paris. Abstr. 17-2-26.

Miller,J.F.A.P. 1961. Immunological function of the thymus. Lancet, 2 : 748-749.

Monier,J.C., Dardenne, M., Pléau,J.M., Schmitt,D., Deschaux,P. and Bach,J.F. 1980. Characterization of FTS in the thymus. I. Fixation of anti-FTS antibodies on thymic reticulo-epithelial cells. Clin.Exp.Immunol., 42 : 470-476.

Pelletier,M., Montplaisir,S., Dardenne,M. and Bach,J.F. 1976. Thymic hormone activity and spontaneous autoimmunity in dwarf mice and their littermates. Immunology, 30 : 783-786.

Pléau,J.M., Pasques,D. and Bach,J.F. 1978. Dosage radioimmunologique du facteur thymique sérique (FTS) in ;"Radioimmunoassay and Related Procedures in Medicine" vol.II. Intern.Atomic Energy Agency, Vienna.

Tubiana,N. and Dardenne,M. 1979. Neonatal thymus graft. I. Studies on the regulation of the level of circulating thymic factor (FTS). Immunology, 36: 207-213.

Twomey,J.J., Goldstein,G., Lewis,V.M., Bealmear,P.M. and Good,R.A. 1977. Bioassay determinations of thymopoietin and thymic hormone levels in human plasma. Proc.Natl.Acad.Sci. (USA), 6: 2541-1545.

Walford,R.L. 1974. Immunologic theory of aging ; current status. Fed. Proc. 33 : 2020-2024.

Zinkernagel,R.M. and Dixon,J.F. 1977. Comparison of T cell-mediated immune responsiveness of NZB, (NZBxNZW)F$_1$ hybrid and other murine strains. Clin.Exp.Immunol. 29: 110-121.

ENHANCED HELPER ACTIVITY IN AGING MICE INJECTED WITH THYMIC FACTORS

Daniela Frasca and Gino Doria

Gruppo di Immunogenetica, Laboratorio di Radiopatologia, C.S.N. Casaccia,

Via Anguillarese km. 1,300, Rome, Italy

ABSTRACT

    The antibody response of carrier-primed spleen cells from old mice, uninjected or injected with thymic factors, has been evaluated in vitro by the Mishell and Dutton technique. The injection of thymic factors has been found to induce a moderate increase in the anti-TNP antibody response only to a T-dependent immunogen as TNP-HRBC. These factors have no effect on the anti-TNP antibody response against TNP-Ficoll, a T-independent immunogen. However, the evidence for T-cell recovery has been only partial, due to the impairment of B-cell reactivity with age. Therefore, the helper activity of carrier-primed spleen cells from old mice, uninjected or injected with thymic factors, has been evaluated by adding graded numbers of these primed cells to cultures containing TNP-HRBC and a constant number of normal spleen cells from young mice. The results from this experimental approach have demonstrated that the thymic factors tested are efficient in the recovery of T-T cell cooperation in the generation of helper activity.

INTRODUCTION

    The antibody response decreases with advancing age. The reduced responsiveness in old animals is associated with defects in B-cell reactivity and in helper T-cell function (Goidl et al., 1976; Krogsrud and Perkins, 1977; Callard and Basten, 1978; Doria et al., 1978; Doria et al., 1980). The involution of the thymus gland, which occurs already from the first weeks of age, is the main cause of the decline in antibody production with age (Hirokawa and Makinodan, 1975). In fact, the concentration of thymic hormones (Bach et al., 1975; Hooper et al., 1975) and the capacity of thymic tissue to influence the differentiation and the maturation of precursor cells into mature T lymphocytes is reduced in old animals. Also in the B-cell population, some defects with age have been described (Callard and Basten, 1978). Unlike lymphocytes, macrophages seem to be unaffected by aging (Callard and Basten, 1978; Perkins, 1971; Heidrick and Makinodan, 1973).

A cellular analysis of age-dependent variations of the in vitro anti body response has been made by techniques suitable to dissect out B and T cell reactivities. 15 month old mice were injected with two different thymic factors to evaluate in vitro their effects on: 1) antibody response of spleen cells to T-dependent and T-independent immunogens and 2) hel per activity of spleen cells from old mice in the antibody response of spleen cells from young mice.

MATERIALS AND METHODS

Animals. Male (C57 Bl/10 x DBA/2) F_1 mice were used at 3 and 15 months of age.

Thymic factors treatment. Synthetic thymic factors, α_1 from Dr. A.L. Goldstein (Goldstein et al., 1977) and the pentapeptide thymopoietin 32-36 from Dr. G. Goldstein (Schlesinger and Goldstein, 1975), were injected i.p.(intraperitoneally) into 15 month old mice (1 or 10 μg/0.2 ml saline/ mouse) over a period of 5 days before carrier-priming.

Carrier-priming. To induce helper activity, mice untreated or treated with thymic factors were injected i.v.(intravenously) with 2×10^5 HRBC (horse red blood cells)/0.2 ml PBS (phosphate buffered saline), 4 days before culture.

In vitro antibody response. The anti-TNP (2,4,6-trinitrophenyl) antibody response to 2×10^5 TNP-HRBC or 2 ng TNP-Ficoll was induced in cultures of 1×10^6 or 1.5×10^6 nucleated spleen cells from HRBC-primed mice, treated or not with thymic factors. Culture conditions have been described previously (Doria et al., 1980). The antibody response was assayed on day 4 and 5, and expressed as number of anti-TNP PFC (plaque-forming cells)/culture.

Titration of helper activity. The helper activity of HRBC-primed spleen cells from treated mice and from untreated age control mice was titrated by a modification of the experimental model of Kettman and Dutton (Mishell and Dutton, 1967). Normal spleen cells cultured alone do not give appreciable anti-TNP/PFC responses, when immunized in vitro with TNP-HRBC. If 1×10^6 normal spleen cells from 3 month old mice were cultu-

red with 2×10^5 TNP-HRBC and graded numbers of spleen cells from HRBC-primed 3 month old mice or 15 month old mice, treated or not with thymic factors, the anti-TNP antibody response increases with the number of primed
spleen cells added. The number of anti-TNP PFC given by 1×10^6 normal
spleen cells was subtracted from the numbers of anti-TNP PFC given by
1×10^6 normal spleen cells supplemented with $5-30 \times 10^4$ HRBC-primed spleen
cells; in this way, the log PFC was a linear function of the log number
of primed cells added. The linear regressions were calculated by the least
squares method. The intercept and slope of these regressions on log-log
scales were used to interpolate curvilinear regressions on linear scales
and to calculate the definite integral value ($PFC \times 10^6$) from 0 to 2×10^5
primed cells added. This integral value was taken as total helper activity.

RESULTS

In the present study, spleen cells from immunodeficient old mice,
injected with thymic factors of synthetic nature, have been evaluated
in vitro for: 1) antibody response against TNP-HRBC and TNP-Ficoll and
2) helper activity of old T cells in the antibody response of young B
cells. The results of one experiment, reported in Table 1, show that the
treatment with thymic factors have been very efficient in the restoration
of helper activity in aged mice. 15 month old mice were left uninjected
or injected daily with 0.2 ml saline containing 1 μg α_1 or 1 μg thymop.
32-36 for 5 consecutive days before carrier-priming. Uninjected 3 month
old mice were used as reference age control. The antibody response of 15
month old mice untreated with thymic factors is about 40% of the response
of 3 month old mice. The decrease in the capacity to mount an antibody
response is due to defects also in B-cell reactivity, as demonstrated by
the results on the variations of the response to TNP-Ficoll, which occur
during the aging process (Doria et al., 1980). However, as shown in the
third column of Table 1, the anti-TNP antibody response of spleen cells
from 15 month old mice injected with α_1 or the pentapeptide is higher
than that yielded by spleen cells from untreated animals, only when

TNP-HRBC has been used as immunogen. In fact, no effect on the response to TNP-Ficoll has been revealed. A more evident effect of the treatment has been observed in a system in which helper T cells from aged, treated mice are added to normal spleen cells from 3 month old mice. The total helper activity values, expressed as $PFCx10^6$, indicate that some changes in the T-cell subpopulations of treated mice have occurred (last column, Table 1). Moreover, these values indicate that α_1 has been more efficient than the pentapeptide.

CONCLUSIONS

The injection of thymic factors into 15 month old mice induces only a moderate increase of the anti-TNP antibody response of their spleen cells to T-dependent immunogens (Table 1, third column; D'Agostaro et al., 1980). This negligeable effect could result from defects in the reactivity of B cells from old mice as well as from a low efficiency of the treatment. However, due to the impairment of B-cell responsiveness in old animals, the evidence for T-cell recovery was only partial. The enhancement in helper activity of spleen cells from old, treated mice was evident from the total helper activity values. Two subpopulations of helper T cells have been found in the spleen of adult mice and named Th1 and Th2; these two cells can synergize in the antibody response by two different mechanisms: the first one recognises the carrier and the second one promotes the polyclonal activation (Tada et al., 1978). It is not yet identified which cell is the target of thymic factors. However, the restoration of helper activity indicates the persistence in old animals of precursor cells which can be stimulated to differentiate into mature T cells. Moreover, even if a stimulatory effect on suppressor T cells cannot be excluded, these thymic factors stimulate T cells to differentiate into helper rather than suppressor cells.

TABLE 1 - RESTORATION OF HELPER ACTIVITY OF HRBC-PRIMED SPLEEN CELLS FROM
OLD MICE INJECTED WITH SYNTHETIC THYMIC FACTORS

Age (months)	Treatment	PFC/culture		Total helper activity (PFC x 10^6)
		TNP-HRBC	TNP-Ficoll	
15	none	195	36	10
15	Thymop. 32-36	455	39	19
15	Thymosin α_1	495	55	27
3	none	515	61	30

REFERENCES

Bach, J.F., Dardenne, M., Pleau, J.M. and Bach, M.A.: Isolation, biochemical characteristics and biological activity of a circulating thymic
hormone in the mouse and in the human. Ann. N.Y. Acad. Sci. 249: 186,
1975.

Callard, R.E. and Basten, A.: Immune functions in aged mice. IV. Loss of T
cell and B cell function in thymus-dependent antibody responses.
Eur. J. Immunol. 8: 552, 1978.

D'Agostaro, G., Frasca, D., Garavini, M. and Doria, G.: Immunorestoration
of old mice by injection of thymus extracts: enhancement of T cell-T
cell cooperation in the in vitro antibody response. Cell. Immunol. 53:
207, 1980.

Doria, G., D'Agostaro, G. and Garavini, M.: Age-dependent changes of B-cell
reactivity and T cell-T cell interaction in the in vitro antibody response. Cell. Immunol. 53: 195, 1980.

Doria, G., D'Agostaro, G. and Poretti, A.: Age-dependent variations of anti
body avidity. Immunol. 35: 601, 1978.

Goidl, E.A., Innes, J.B. and Weksler, M.E.: Immunological studies of aging.
II. Loss of IgG and high avidity plaque-forming cells and increased
suppressor cell activity in aging mice. J. Exp. Med. 144: 1037, 1976.

Goldstein, A.L., Low, T.L.K., Mc Adoo, M., Mc Clure, J., Thurman, J.B.,
Rossio, J., Laj, C.Y., Chang, D., Wang, S.S., Harvey, C., Ramel, A.H.
and Meienhofer, J.: Thymosin α_1: isolation and sequence analysis of an
immunologically active polypeptide. Proc. Nat. Acad. Sci. 74: 725,
1977.

Heidrick, M.L. and Makinodan, T.: Presence of impairment of humoral immunity in nonadherent spleen cells of old mice. J. Immunol. 111: 1502,
1973.

Hirokawa, K. and Makinodan, T.: Thymic involution: effect on T cell differentiation. J. Immunol. 114: 1659, 1975.

Hooper, J.A., Mc Daniel, M.C., Thurman, G.B., Cohen, G.H., Schulof, R.S. and Goldstein, A.L.: Purification and properties of bovine thymosin. Ann. N.Y. Acad. Sci. 249: 125, 1975.

Krogsrud, R.L. and Perkins, E.H.: Age-related changes in T cell function. J. Immunol. 118: 1607, 1977.

Mishell, R.I. and Dutton, R.W.: Immunization of dissociated spleen cell cultures from normal mice. J. Exp. Med. 126: 423, 1967.

Perkins, E.H.: Phagocytic activity of aged mice. J. Reticuloendoth. 9: 642, 1971.

Schlesinger, D.H. and Goldstein, G.: The amino acid sequence of thymopoietin II. Cell. 5: 361, 1975.

Tada, T., Takemori, T., Okumura, K., Nonaka, M. and Tokuhisa, T.: Two distinct types of helper T cells involved in the secondary antibody response: independent and synergistic effects of Ia^- and Ia^+ helper T cells. J. Exp. Med. 147: 446, 1978.

THYROID-DEPENDENCE OF AGE-RELATED DECLINE OF FTS PRODUCTION

N. Fabris, E. Mocchegiani and M. Muzzioli.

Immunol. Ctr., INRCA Res. Dept.

Ancona, ITALY

ABSTRACT

The progressive decline with advancing age of the circulating level of FTS (facteur thymique serique) depends both on intrinsic and extrinsic factors. Among the microenviromental factors, the age-dependent alteration of thyroid hormone turnover seems to play a major role. Short-term treatment of old mice with L-thyroxine restores the production of FTS and increases both the number of RFCs and the PHA response. The action of thyroxine is exerted through the recipient thymus, since it is uneffective in athymic nude mice.

INTRODUCTION

It has been suggested that the age-dependent decline of the immunological vigor may be due either to intrinsic factors, impairing the "old" lymphocytes from reacting to physiological stimuli with the appropriate response, or to extrinsic factors, primarely related to the microenviroment which should sustain the immune response (Makinodan, 1977).

This last view has been furtherly supported by the demonstration that many enviromental factors doubtlessly act on the efficiency of the lymphoid cells (Fabris, 1981). Among these factors a primary relevance has been assigned to neuro-endocrine humoral factors, which in a number of different experimental models have been proven to modulate the immune response (Fabris, 1977).

If the action of these factors is substantially supported by a good body of experimental evidence, their mechanism of action is at present not yet well defined; while it is out of doubt that they can act directly on mature lymphocytes, since receptors for hormones or neurotransmitters have been proven to exist on their membrane surface, it cannot be excluded that other mechanisms may be involved as well.

It has been, for istance, demonstrated that the differentiation and maturation of the lymphoid system is under the influence of humoral factors produced by the thymus (Goldstein et al., 1977) and, on the other

hand, that microenviromental factors may exert their action also on the
rate of synthesis and/or release of such factors (Bach and Beaurain,
1979).

It is, therefore, hypothyzeable that the age-related decline of immu
nological vigor might well depend on the progressive reduction of the en
docrine activity of the thymus (Weksler et al., 1978) and that such a re
duction might be caused, to a certain extent, by age-associated alterations of those microenviromental factors which physiologically modulate
the turnover of thymic factors (Fabris et al., in press).

Among the microenviromental factors which may be relevant in this
context it is out of doubt that hormones and neurotransmitters play a ma
jor role. This assumption is supported by two orders of considerations:
firstly, that it is unlikely that an endocrine activity, such as that re
presented by the secretion of thymic factors might work in the complete
ly autonomous manner thus far proposed; secondly that with advancing age
consistent alterations do affect the body homeostatic mechanisms, causing
either modifications on the rate of synthesis and/or release of various
hormones and neurotransmitters (Andres and Tobin, 1977) or changes in the
sensitivity of target cells to their action (Roth and Adelman, 1975).

Since one of the most frequent homeostatic changes observed in advan
ced age consists in a decreased function of thyroid hormones (Herrman et
al., 1981), we have investigated whether short-term treatment of old mice
with thyroxine may reactivate the nearly absent production of thymic factors observed in old individuals and, consequently, recover the deficient
peripheral immune response. These data have been compared to those ones
obtained in old mice grafted with a neonatal thymus. Furthermore, in order to determine whether the action of thyroxine is directly exerted on
the thymus, hormonal treatment has been also performed in athymic nude
mice.

MATERIALS AND METHODS.

Animals: male Balb/c mice used in these experiments, were housed in
plastic cages and fed with pelletted food and water ad libitum. The mana
gement of these animals for long periods of time includes also smallpox
vaccination at 2 months of age and 4 day tetracycline (Pfitzer) treatment in the drinking water 4 times a year. In our housing conditions the

life-span of Balb/c mice ranges between 24 and 28 months.

Body weight of experimental animals was determined at the beginning and at the end of each experiment and percentual variations evaluated.

Thymus_graft: thymus graft was implanted under the Kidney capsule in anesthetized mice. Successfull implantation was assessed at sacrifice.

Thyroxine_preparation_and_injection_schedule: L-thyroxine (Fluka) was dissolved in a small volume of alcalinized water (pH 7.8-8.0) and saline was then added to reach the final concentration. Daily subcutaneous injections were made between 9.00 and 11.00 a.m.. The day of sacrifice, animals did not receive thyroxine injections.

Mitogen_responses: Spleen cells from unimmunized mice, obtained by teasing the spleens through a 60 seave, were washed twice in Hank's solution, counted and resuspended to a final concentration of $3x10^6$ trypan-blue excluding cells/ml, in RPMI (Eurobio-France) additioned with glutamine, antibiotics (Eurobio) and 5% fresh inactivated male human serum. Aliquots of 0, 1ml were distributed in microwells (Cook). Mitogens were then added in the amount of 10 ul/well. After incubation at 37°C in a CO_2 atmosphere for 48 hr, 1 uCi of H^3-thymidine (Amershan, specific activity 5000 mC/mM) was added to each well. Cells were collected 20 hrs later, by an automatic cell-harvester (Skatron, Norway) and radio-activity determined by a scintillation counter (Tricarb-Packard). Triplicate cultures were prepared for each mitogen concentration. Phytohaemagglutinin M (PHA, Difco) was used at two different final concentrations: 0.05 and 0.0125 ml^{-1}. Concanavallin-A (Con-A, Serva) was used at the final concentrations of 30 and 7.5 ug/ml. Lypopolysaccaride (LPS from E. Coli, Difco) was used at the final concetrations of 160 and 40 ug/ml.

Facteur_thymique_serique_ (FTS) determination: The FTS activity has been measured according to Bach procedure (Bach et Dardenne, 1972) with minor modifications. Briefly plasma samples have been filtered through a Centriflo Amicon membranes with a cut-off of 50.000 daltons. 50 ul of the filtrate or of serial dilution of it made with Hank's solution were mixed with 200 ul of spleen cell suspension from thymectomized mice (final suspension $=7.5 \cdot 10^6$ cells/ml) and incubated at 37° C for 3'.

After washing, cells were resuspended in 250 ul of a solution of Aza
thioprine (Wellcome) at the concentration of 10 ug/ml, incubated at 37° C
for 60', after which 250 ul of a sheep red blood cells suspension containing $12.5 \cdot 10^6$ cells/ml were added. After a further 5' incubation at 37° C,
cells were centrifuged in the cold at 100 xG for 5', resuspended for 5'
by using a rotating system (10 cm diameter, 8 rev./min.) and counted in
an hemocytometer chanber. The rosette forming cells (RFCs) present in
18.000 spleen cells have been counted and values recorded as $RFCs/1 \cdot 10^6$
cells. The titre of FTS was considered as the maximal dilution still able
to induce Azathioprine sensitivity in 50% of the number of RFCs recorded
in control cells.

Determination of rosette-forming-cells (RFC): RFCs have been determined according to Bach procedure (Bach and Dardenne, 1972). Spleen cells
to be assayed for RFC capacity have been treated with Azathioprine or
Hank's solution, with the same technique reported for FTS determination.

RESULTS

A. Recovery of immunological efficiency by neonatal thymus graft.
    Table I shows the effect of a neonatal thymus graft, performed in old
mice, on different immunological parameters. Both the number of Rosette-

TABLE I. Recovery of age-related immune deficiencies by neonatal thymus
          graft or short-term thyroxine treatment.

Experimental Group	Serum FTS activity (Log_2 of reciprocal of titre)	No. of RFC $/1 \cdot 10^6$ spleen cells.	No. of AZA-insensitive $RFC/1 \cdot 10^6$ spleen c.	PHA response (mitotic index)
Young	5.82 ± 0.50	977 ± 51	356 ± 58	24.4 ± 2.0
Old	1.32	598 ± 49	253 ± 59	10.8 ± 2.2
Old+Thymus	5.32 ± 0.10	862 ± 51	345 ± 30	18.4 ± 3.1
Old+Thyroxine	3.57 ± 0.25	920 ± 26	329 ± 14	20.5 ± 3.2

-forming-cells and the mitogen resonse to phytohaemagglutinin by spleen
cells, which are abnormally low in old mice, are recovered by a neonatal
thymus graft to values comparable in young mice. Concomittantly, also the

160

circulating level of FTS, which is virtually absent in the sera of old mi
ce, is reconstituted to the values observed in young mice. Experiments
not reported here, have demonstrated that the recovery of all these parameters does not occur with the same Kinetics: rosette-formation and FTS
level are recovered few days after neonatal thymus graft, whereas reconstitution of mitogen response requires two to three weeks.

B.   Recovery of immunological efficiency by thyroxine treatment.

Treatment with 15 daily injections with thyroxine at the dose of 0.1
ug/g body weight/day is able to recover the immunological efficiency of
old mice in a fashion quite similar to that observed after grafting with
a neonatal thumus (Table I). Also in this case, in fact, FTS activity appears again in the sera of old animals, followed by reconstitution of ro
sette-forming-capacity and of PHA response.

C.   Effect of neonatal thymus graft or thyroxine treatment in athymic nu-
     de mice.

As reported in Table II, nude mice show, as expected, an absent level of FTS activity, a lack of Azathioprine sensitive rosette-forming-

TABLE II.   Uneffectiveness of short-term thyroxine treatment in resto-
            ring the immune deficiencies of athymic nude mice.

Experimental Groups	Serum FTS activity (Log_2 of reciprocal of titre).	No. of RFC $/1 \cdot 10^6$ sple en cells.	No. of AZA-insensitive RFC/$1 \cdot 10^6$ spleen c.	PHA re-sponse (mitotic index).
Young	5.42 ± 0.45	1.050 ± 48	570 ± 52	26.0 ± 3.0
Nude	1.32 ± 0.10	734 ± 46	652 ± 43	2.3 ± 0.4
Nude+Thymus	3.82 ± 0.50	980 ± 65	530 ± 60	21.5 ± 3.6
Nude+Thyroxine	1.32 ± 0.10	672 ± 61	576 ± 39	2.9 ± 0.5

cells (T-rosette) and an irrelevant response to PHA. By grafting a neonatal thymus into nude mice all these parameters are corrected.

By contrast treatment of nude mice with thyroxine is totally incapable to recover any one of the immune functions taken into consideration.

DISCUSSION

From the data reported in the present paper, the following general
considerations can be made: a) with advancing age a significant decline of
FTS production is observed in Balb/c mice; b) a neonatal thymus graft is
able to restore the FTS level in old mice and concomittantly to reconstitute the low number of rosette-forming-cells and the abnormal PHA response; c) similar reconstitution is achieved in old mice by a short-term
treatment with L-thyroxine; d) a neonatal thymus graft, but not thyroxine
treatment is able to recover both FTS level and peripheral immune efficiency in athymic nude mice.

The causes of the age-related immunological decline have been primarely related to the precociousness in life of the involution of the thymus, as producer either of mature T-cells (Makinodan, 1977) and/or of
thymic humoral factors (Bach and Beaurain, 1979). In both cases it is, ho
wever, controversial whether the nature of such an age-dependent deterio
ration is due to intrinsic or extrinsic factors and whether this altera
tion is to some extent reversible.

Our data on the effectiveness of thyroxine treatment to correct the
age-related decline of different immunological functions, clearly support
the assumption that microenviromental factors play a considerable role in
the ageing of the immune system.

In our experimental model one of the earliest modifications induced
by thyroxine treatment is the appeatance of detectable FTS levels, and
the increment of the number of T-rosettes, which is strictly linked to
the FTS level itself. The recovery of the other immunological parameters
is somewhat delayed.

Regardless these considerations, it is to be stressed the point that,
according to our (Fabris et al., in press) and other authors findings
(Pelletier, et al., 1976) also the endocrine activity of the thymus depends to large extent, on microenviromental factors and primarely on the
neuro-endocrine balance.

That the action of thyroxine is exerted at this level is furtherly sup
ported by the fact that its restoring effect on the immune efficiency is
not observable in nude mice, thus suggesting that the presence of the thy
mus is essential in order to allow thyroxine to exert its effects.

In this context it is necessary, however, to remind that, on the one
hand, with advancing age the whole neuroendocrine system shows a number
of alterations related either to the secretion rate of hormones or to the
responsiveness of peripheral tissues (Roth and Adelman, 1975), and, on the
other hand, that the action of thyroid hormones themselves, may require

the cooperation of other hormones, as suggested by the strict relationships exsting between them and the autonomous nervous system (Brodie et
al., 1969).

Finally, it should be taken in mind that thyroxine may act also directly on peripheral mature cells, turning them from an unresponsive state
to a more physiological condition. That such a modification might take
place is supported by the fact that lymphocytes possess receptors for
both T_3 and T_4, although it is yet unknown whether they are expressed on
the surface of all different lymphocyte subpopulations (Lemarchand-Beraud
et al., 1977).

References

Andres, R. and Tobin, J.D., 1977. Endocrine systems, In: Finch, C.E. and
    Hayflick, L. (Eds), Handbook of the biology of aging. Van Mostrand-
    Reinhold, New York, 357.
Bach, J.F., Dardenne, M., Papiernik, M., Barvis, A., Levasseur, P. and
    Lebrand, H., Evidence for a serum-factor secreted by the human thymus
    Lancet, 2, 1056, 1972.
Bach, J.F., and Beaurain, G., 1979. Role òf intrinsic and extrinsic fac-
    tors in FTS production. J. Immunol., 122, 2505.
Brodie, B.B., Daviea, J.J., Hynie, S., Krishna, G. and Weiss, B., 1969.
    Interrerelationship of catecholamines with other endocrine systems,
    Pharmacol. Rev., 18, 273.
Fabris, N., Piantanelli, L. and Muzzioli, M., 1977. Differential effect
    of pregnancy or gestanges on humoral and cell-mediated immunity, Clin.
    Exp. Immunol., 28, 306.
Fabris, N., Mocchegiani, E., and Muzzioli, M.. Functional interactions
    between the neuroendocrine balance and FTS production. In: N. Fabris
    E. Garaci, and N.A. Mitchison (Eds) Immunoregulation 1981. Plenum
    Press.. (in press).
Fabris, N., 1981. Body Homeostatic mechanisms and ageing of immune system.
    In: T. Makinodan and M.M.B. Kay (Eds) "Immunology and aging". CRC
    Press Palm Beach, (in press).
Goldstein, A.L., Low, T.L.K., McAdoo, M., McGlure, J., Thurman, G.B., Ros-
    sio, J., Lai, C.Y., Chang, D., Wang, S.S., Harvey, C., Ramel, A.H.,
    Meienhofer, J., 1977.. Thymosin: isolation and sequence analysis of
    an immunologically active thymic polyptide, Proc. Natl. Acad. Sci.,
    74, 725.
Hermann, J., Heinen, E., Kröll, H.J., Rudorff, K.H. and Krüskemper, H.L.,
    1981. Low T_3 Syndrome in old Age. In: R-D Hesch (Ed.) The "Low T_3
    Syndrome", 249.
Lemarcand-Beraud, T., Holm, A.C. and Scazziga, B.R., 1977. Triiodo-thyro-
    nine and thyroxine nuclear receptors in lymphocytes from normal, hy-
    per and hypothyroid patients, Act. Endocrinol., 85, 44.
Makinodan, T., Good, R.A., and Kay, M.M.B., 1977. Cellular basic of immu-
    nosenescence, in: Makinodan, T., and Yunis, E., (Eds). Comprehensive
    Immunology N° 1 Plenum Press., N.Y., 9.
Pellettier, M., Montplaisir, S., Dardenne, M., Bach, J.F., 1976. Thymic
    hormone activity and spontaneous autoimmunity in dwarf mice and their
    littermates, Immunology, 30, 783.
Roth, G.S., and Adelman, R.C., 1975. Age-related changes in hormone bin-
    ding by target cells and tissues: Possible role in altered adaptive
    responsiveness, Exp. Gerontol., 10, 1.
Weksler, M.E., Innes, J.B., Goldstein, G., 1978. Immunological studies
    of aging IV. The contribution of thymic involution to the immune defi
    ciencies of aging mice and reversal with thymopoietin. J. Exp. Med.
    148, 996-1006.

SESSION V

IMMUNE DISFUNCTIONS IN AGED HUMANS.

IMMUNE SENESCENCE IN MAN

Marc L. Weksler, M. D.
Department of Medicine
Cornell University Medical College
New York, N.Y. 10021
U. S. A.

ABSTRACT
   This review attempts to place in perspective a large body of knowledge concerning immune senescence. My approach is to discuss in detail results of clinical studies, using studies involving experimental animals to extend and amplify conclusions drawn from investigation in man. The working hypothesis that serves as the basis of this review is that the involution of the thymus gland after sexual maturity plays a critical role in the senescence of the immune system.

THYMIC INVOLUTION AND AGING

   The involution of the thymus gland after puberty was recognized long before the immunologic function of this gland was discovered. In the early 1930's careful anatomical studies showed that the mass of the human thymus gland, well maintained until 15 years of age, rapidly shrank after sexual maturity (Boyd, 1932). By the age of 45 or 50 the lymphoid mass of the human thymus is only 15% of its maximal mass. Thirty years later, in the early 1960's an immunological function of the thymus was first recognized. Today the crucial role of the thymus in humoral and cell mediated immunity, and in the regulation of the immune response is well established. It is logical, therefore, to consider the contribution of thymic involution to the changes in the immune system observed with aging.

   The major function of the thymus gland is to export a subpopulation of lymphocytes. The thymic-derived lymphocytes (T lymphocytes) arise in the bone marrow and migrate to the thymus where their differentiation continues. Although the differentiation process is not completely understood, it is known that the microenvironment of the gland as well as hormones produced by the gland are important in the maturation of T lymphocytes. After sexual maturity, the thymus begins to involute and loses its capacity to facilitate the differentiation of pre-thymic T cell precursors.

One marker of T cell maturation, acquired in the thymus, is the receptor for sheep erythrocytes. The presence of this receptor has offered a convenient method to enumerate T lymphocytes. Mature T-lymphocytes form "rosettes" with sheep erythrocytes. The age-associated decline in the capacity of the human thymus to stimulate the maturation of T lymphocytes is manifested by the decreasing percentage of T cells within the thymus that bind sheep erythrocytes with age. Thus, 85 per cent of the thymic lymphocytes at the age of 20 bind sheep erythrocytes. This number falls to 65 per cent at 50 years of age and 50 per cent at 80 years of age (Singh and Singh, 1979).

The progressive decline in the capacity of the thymus gland to mediate lymphoid differentiation has also been demonstrated by transplantation studies in experimental animals. Thumus glands from mice of different ages have been transplanted into young, syngeneic, thymectomized recipients (Hirokawa and Makinodan, 1975). Thymus glands from oldest donors were least able to mediate the differentiation of T cell precursors. Thymus glands from newborn to 3 month old mice were most effective. Thymus glands taken from animals more than three months of age showed a progressive loss in their capacity to reconstitute theta positive T cells in the peripheral lymphoid organs or to reconstitute thymic-dependent immune function.

The influence of the thymus on lymphocyte maturation had been thought to be limited to the T lymphocyte subpopulation. Recently, the thymus has also been found to play a crucial role in the maturation of B lymphocytes (Szewczuk, DeKruff, Weksler and Siskind, 1980). The capacity of B-lymphocytes to generate a normal heterogeneous response with respect to affinity depends on exposure to thymocytes. The age of the thymocytes determines their capacity to bring about this maturation of B lymphocytes. Thus, thymocytes from mice more than six months of age are severly impaired in their capacity to mediate B cell maturation compared with the capacity of thymocytes from 1 or 2 month old mice.

During the past ten years several putative thymic hormones (thymopoietin, thymosin, facteur thymique serique) have been isolated, purified, and
the amino acid sequence of several determined. The serum concentration of
each of these hormones has been shown to decline with age. Thymopoietin levels in human serum are well maintained between birth and thirty years of
age. Thereafter, there is a linear decline in serum thymopoietin activity.
No activity was found in healthy humans over the age of 60 years (Lewis,
Twomey, Bealmear, Goldstein and Good, 1978). The concentration of FTS in hu
man serum begins to fall after the age of 20 and becomes undetectable after
the age of 50 (Bach, Papiernik, Levasseur, Dardenne, Barois and Brigand,
1972). The concentration of thymosin alpha 1 in human serum appears to decline even earlier.

Despite the involution of the thymus gland, the number of peripheral T
cells does not change significantly with age. Most studies have shown that
the relative and absolute number of human T lymphocytes in the blood of humans does not change between the ages of 20 and 90 years (Gupta and Good,
1979). Similar studies in normal long lived mice have also shown that the
number of splenic T-lymphocytes does not change with age (Stutman, 1972).
However, in short-lived autoimmune prone mice an age-associated decrease
in the number of T lymphocytes in the spleen was reported. It is possible
that aged humans with autoantibodies have fewer T cells than normal.

The maintenance of a normal number of T cells with age despite the involution of the thymus gland and the decline in the serum concentration of
thymic hormones may appear paradoxical. However, it is important to appreciate that the number of T cells depends not only on T cell production but
on T cell destruction. As T cells appear to be extremely long-lived cells
it is possible that residual thymic function present during middle and old
age is sufficient to replace the small number of T cells that are destro-
yed. It should also be rembered that the total T cell population has not
been measured. Usually, only one, the blood or spleen, of a number of lymphoid compartements is sampled and the T-cell complement in this compartment
found to be unchanged with age. It remains a definite possibility that the

total number of T cells within the body of young and old individuals is
different.

SENESCENCE OF THE IMMUNE RESPONSE

The effect of age on immunity was first noted more than 50 years ago
when the serology of human blood groups substances was being studied. The
serum concentration of antibody to the human erytrocyte A and B antigens,
was found to decline with age (Thomsen and Kettel, 1929). Subsequently, an
tibody levels of humans to the thymic dependent antigen, sheep erythrocytes, was also found to decline with age (Paul and Bunnel, 1932). The highest levels of anti-sheep erythrocyte antibody were found in individuals
between the ages of 15 and 20 years. Subsequently, there was a progressive
decline in the titer of this antibody with age. More recently, the effect
of age on the immune response of humans to salmonella flagellin was measured (Roberts-Thompson, et. al., 1974). Old individuals produced less IgG
anti-flagellin antibody than did young individuals. In contrast, to the de
cline in these antibodies to foreign antigens observed with age the level
of autoantibodies is higher in older than in young individuals (Hallgren,
et. al., 1973). As we shall note throughout this review, an important gene
ralization drawn from the study of immune senescence is the decreased immune response to foreign antigens and the increased response to self antigens with age. Despite the decreased immune response to foreign antigens
with age, there is no decline in the serum concentration of immunoglobulin
(Hallgren, et. al., 1973). It is possible that the decreased antibody response to foreign antigens is balanced by the increased antibody response
to autologous antigens. In this way total immunoglobulin concentration may
be maintained.

A decrease in the antibody response to foreign antigens and an increa
se in autoantibodies has also been observed as experimental animals age.
Thus, the response of mice to sheep erythrocytes falls with age while the
level of antinuclear antibody rises with age (Singhal, Roder and Duwe,
1979). These findings suggest that the characteristic age-associated de-

fect in immune competence reflects not only a deficiency of thymic function but in addition an altered regulation of immune function.

The decline in thymic-dependent immunity affects not only the antibody
response to most antigens but also delayed cutaneous hypersensitivity, tumor and graft rejection, and resistance to myco-bacterial, viral and fungal
infection. Delayed cutaneous hypersensitivity to a variety of antigens has
been tested in humans of various ages (Roberts-Thompson, et.al., 1974).Sub
jects over the age of 60 were significantly impaired in their delayed cuta
neous reactivity. A lower percentage of humans over the age of 70, compared
with subjects less than 70, have positive skin reactions to tuberculin (Wal
ford, Willkens and Decker, 1968). The loss of T-cell mediated immunity to
mycobacterium tuberculosis probably contributes to the clinical observation
that reactivation tuberculosis is seen with increasing frequency among the
elderly. The loss of delayed cutaneous hypersensitivity is not due solely
to a loss of immunological memory resulting from the long time between sen
sitization and immune challenge. When young and old humans were sensitized
for the first time with dinitrochlorobenzene (DNCB) and challenged a short
time later only 5% of subjects less than 70 years of age could not be sensitized to DNCB, while 30% of the subjects over 70 could not be sensitized
(Walford, Willkens and Decker, 1968).

The impaired antibody response and delayed cutaneous hypersensitivity
observed in these clinical studies did not distinguish between a primary
defect in the immune system or a failure of the environment of the elderly
host to support a normal immune response. This question was examined by
studying the response of lymphocytes from old humans in vitro, and by studying the behavior of lymphocytes from older experimental animals after
transfer to young animals. Under these circumstances the intrinsic activity of lymphocytes can be measured free of other physiological changes that
accompany aging, which may compromise immune functions within the old host.
T-lymphocytes from sensitized humans proliferate when cultured with antigen.
As the cutaneous response to PPD was impaired with age, it was important to
know if the lymphocyte response of old humans to PPD was impaired. The pro-

liferative response of lymphocytes from patients with tuberculosis was mea‐
sured in cultures with PPD (Nilsson, 1971). Lymphocytes from old patients
incorporated less thymidine in culture with PPD than did lymphocytes from
young patients. The proliferative response of T-lymphocytes was inverserly
correlated with age. Thus, an intrinsic defect in the function of T-lympho‐
cytes from old persons was demonstrated. The proliferative response of T-
lymphocytes from old humans stimulated by the plant lectins, phytohemagglu‐
tinin (PHA) and pokeweed mitogen (PWM) or by allogeneic or autologous non
T-lymphocytes is also impaired (Weksler and Hutteroth, 1974; Fernandez and
MacSween, 1980).

The cellular basis of the age-associated defect in human T cell proli‐
feration has been studies in detail (Inkeles, et al., 1977). Although the
total number of T cells is the same in old and young humans, there are on‐
ly one half the number of mitogen-responsive T cells in the blood of old
subjects as in young subjects. This conclusion was based upon three inde‐
pendent assays. The number of mitogen responsive T-cells were determined
by limiting dilution analysis, by susceptibility to viral infection and by
thymidine incorporation in the presence of colchicine. There was no diffe‐
rence in the capacity of T cells from old or young subjects to interact
with PHA. Thus, the number and affinity of lymphocyte receptors for PHA
was the same in T cell preparations from young and old subjects.

Not only were the number of mitogen-responsive T cells reduced in old
donors but the capacity of mitogen responsive T cells to divide repeate‐
dly in culture was impaired (Hefton, Darlington, Casazza and Weksler,1980).
This was shown by measuring the number of lymphocytes dividing for the
first, second or third time after 72 hours in culture with PHA. Although
the number of cells dividing for the first time after 72 hours with PHA was
comparable in cultures from old or from young donors, the number of T cells
from old donors dividing for a second or third time was only-half or one-
-quarter of the number of T cells dividing a second or third time, respec‐
tively, in cultures from young donors. This defect in the proliferative ca‐
pacity of lymphocytes from old donors is similar to the defect in the pro‐

liferative response of other cells from old humans. Thus, fibroblasts (Martin, Sprague and Epstein, 1970) and arterial smooth cells (Bierman, 1978) from old humans divide fewer times in culture than do fibroblasts or arterial smooth muscle cells obtained from young persons.

The molecular basis of the proliferative defect observed in old humans has been investigated. Recent studies indicate that a T cell product, T-cell growth factor, secreted during culture is the driving force behind T cell proliferation. The production of T cell growth factor by lymphocytes from young and old humans has been compared (Gillis, Kozak, Durante and Weksler, 1981). Lymphocytes from old humans were found to produce only 50% as much T cell growth factor in culture as do lymphocytes from young donors. Not only do lymphocytes from old humans produce less T cell growth factor but they do not respond to this factor. Thus, T cell growth factor which stimulates the proliferation of T cells from young persons do not stimulate the proliferation of T cells from old persons. This appears to be due, at least in part, to a failure of lymphocytes from old donors to bind T cell growth factor. Whether this is due to a decrease is the number and/or affinity of receptors for T cell growth factor has not be determined.

Prostaglandins are other regulatory molecules which have been implicated in the impaired proliferative response of lymphocytes from old donors. T-lymphocytes from old donors appear to be more sensitive to the inhibitory effects of the prostaglandins of the E series produced in culture by blood monocytes (Goodwin and Messner, 1979). This thesis was supported by the observation that indomethacin which blocks prostaglandin synthesis, augments the proliferative response of T-lymphocytes from old donors. The greatest augmentation was observed in lymphocytes cultures from donors which were most impaired in the absence of indomethacin. It has also been reported that macrophages from old individuals may secrete more prostaglandin of the series than macrophages from young donors (Rosenstein and Strausser, 1980).

Recently techniques have been developed to measure antibody production

by human lymphocytes in culture. Both T dependent and T independent antibo
dy synthesis can be stimulated by formalinized staphylococci in culture.
Using this assay an age associated defect in antibody production in human
lymphocytes in culture has been found (Kim, Siskind and Weksler, 1980).
When these responses were measured in humans of different ages, staphylococci were found to induce significantly fewer PFC in unfractionated lymphocyte preparations from old humans subjects than from young subjects.Ho-
wever, there was no significant difference in the PFC response of purified
B-lymphocyte preparations from old or young subjects cultured with staphylococci. More PFC were generated in culture from young donors containing
unfractioned lymphocytes than in cultures containing B lymphocytes. In con
trast, more PFC were generated in cultures containing lymphocytes. These
results suggest that the age-associated immune defect resides predominantly in the non B-lymphocytes preparation. The non-B cell preparation augments the B cell response in the young but suppresses the response in the
aged. The conclusion that B-lymphocytes from old humans were little affected by aging was supported by studies which showed that the proliferative
response of B-lymphocytes from young or old donors was comparable. Thus,
thymidine incorporation by B-lymphocytes incubated with either staphylococ
ci or anti-human Ig antibody was comparable in B lymphocyte preparation from
young or old humans.

   The function of macrophages in the immune response has been difficult
to evaluate. The recent finding that the addition of lipopolysaccharide to
human macrophages stimulates, the release of a factor which replaces murine T cells in the primary antibody response of murine B cells cultured
with sheep erythrocytes, has offered an assay of human macrophage function.
The capacity of macrophages from old and young humans to produce this T-
cell replacing factor has been measured (Kim, Siskind and Weksler, 1980).
Macrophages from either old or young humans produced an active T cell replacing factor which reconstituted the PFC response of murine B cells. These studies suggest the human macrophages like human B-lymphocytes from old
donors are not significantly impaired with age. The predominant defect in

immune function of lymphocytes from old humans appears to reside in the T-lymphocyte population. T cell function is altered in two ways by age:impaired response to T cell stimuli and suppression by T cells of B-cell responses.

The immunobiology of aging has also been extensively studied in mice. The availability of inbred strains of mice has permitted genetic analysis of lifespan and immune senescence. In addition, inbred strains of mice permit lymphocyte transfer studies which are not possible in the outbred human species. The fact that different species, and strains within species, vary in their lifespan indicate a genetic control of aging. Until recently little was known about the number or location of genes that regulate lifespan. Theoretical interpretation of paleontological evidence of changes in the lifespan of man suggested that relatively few genes (less than a thousand) regulate lifespan (Cutler, 1975). In mice, some of the genes that regulate lifespan are located in the major histocompatibility complex. This is relevant to immune senescence as the major histocompatibility complex contains genes than regulate the immune response. Congenic mice, identical except for small segments in the major histocompatibility complex have different maximal lifespan (Smith and Walford, 1977). Furthermore, mice with the longest lifespan have the longest preserved immune competence. This suggests that genes within the major histocompatibility complex not only modulate lifespan but such genes also influence the rate of immune senescence.

Immune senescence had been demonstrated in mice by a decline of the antibody response to the T dependent antigen, sheep erythrocytes, with age. More recently, the immune deficiency associated with aging in the mouse has been characterized in greater detail by measuring the antihapten PFC response of mice of different ages immunized with the T dependent antigen dinitrophenylated bovine gamma globulin (DNP-BGG) (Goidl, Innes and Weksler, 1976). Although the total antibody response decreases with age, there is a preferential loss od high affinity and IgG anti DNP antibody in old mice. This finding has potential implications both for the health of old animals and for the mechanism underlying immune senescence. High affinity antibody probably effords more protection to infection than low affinity antibody. Thus, the increased suceptibility of old animals to infection may reflect, in part, the loss of high affinity antibody production. As a number of antigen receptors must be engaged to activate lymphocytes, the affinity of antigen receptors is crucial to the immune response. If the affinity of antigen receptors for antigen decreases, more antigen is required to activate the cell. The loss of high affinity lymphocytes probably explains the observation that a higher dose of antigen is necessary to elicit maximal immune re sponse in old as compared to in young animals (Makinodan and Adler, 1975). Of course, if more antigen is required to initiate an immune response, infectious disease would progress further before host resistance develops. Loss of high affinity lymphocytes probably also explains the observation that increased doses of tolerogen are required to induce tolerance in old animals. Furthermore, low concentrations of autologous antigens which may be sufficient to maintain self-tolerance in young animals may not maintain self-tolerance in old animals. The loss of self-tolerance in old animals may result in the increased frequency of auto antibodies in old animals.

The production of high affinity and IgG antibody depends upon normal thymic function. As thymic function wanes with age, the loss of high affinity and IgG antibody with age can be directly related to the involution of the thymus gland. This conclusion is supported by the finding that the loss of high affinity and IgG antibody with age is accelerated by removing the thymus gland and the finding that old mice given the thymic hormone, thymopoietin, regain their capacity to make IgG and high affinity antibody (Weksler, Innes and Goldstein, 1978). The primacy of thymic involution in immune senescence is also supported by the finding that, in general, the immune response to T-independent antigens is less affected than the response to T-dependent antigens (Makinodan and Adler, 1975). The response of so me T-independent antigens is unchangable (Weksler, Innes and Goldstein, 1978) with age while the response to other thymic independent antigen declines (Gallard, Basten and Waters, 1977) with age. Whether the observed changes in the response to T-independent antigens reflect an intrinsic defect in B cell function or extrinsic effect on B cells secondary to increa sed suppressor T cell activity or failure of the thymus gland in old animals to mediate B cell maturation is not always clear.

The cellular basis of the age-associated defects in lymphocyte function in experimental animals has also been investigated in vitro. In addition, transfer studies, not possible in humans, have provided additional insights into the immune deficiency of aging. In such studies, the reactivity of lymphocytes from old or from young animals are compared after their transfer to syngeneic, lethally-irradiated, young receipients. This technique permits a direct assessment of in vivo immune function of lympho cytes from old or young mice free of the influence of age-associated physiological or pathological changes that may occur in old animals.

The response of murine lymphocytes from old animals in vitro has confirmed the results of the human studies. Thus, the response of T-lymphocy tes from old mice to plant lectins or allogeneic lymphocytes declines with age (Adler and Chrest, 1979). This is due, as we found in man, to a decline in the number of mitogen-responsive T cells and to an impaired capacity of the mitogen-responsive cells to divide repeatedly in culture. Other T cell functions studies in vitro, the generation of cytotoxic T-cells in mixed lymphocyte cultures and the generation of graft-versus-host reactions, also decline with age.

A primary, specific PFC response to both T dependent and T independent antigens can be generated in cultures of murine spleen cells. The in vi tro PFC response to the T-dependent antigen, sheep erythocytes, has been extensively studies and has been found to be markedly impaired with age (DeKruff, Kim, Siskind and Weksler, 1980). By 18 months of age Balb/c mi ce retain less than 10% of the maximal PFC response observed between the ages of 3 and 6 months. Several age-associated immune defects contribute to the impaired PFC responses to sheep erythrocytes. Thus, deficiency of helper T-cells, excessive suppressor T cell activity as well as defects in B cell function have been demonstrated. Evidence for an intrinsic age-associated defect in B cell function was found by measuring the anti-DNP-PFC response of spleen cells cultured with DNP-polyacrylamide beads. In these experiments, the B cell response was impaired despite the removal of T cells from the cultured spleens showing that the effect was not due to a suppressive effect of non-B lymphocytes. The proliferative response of B lymphocytes in culture has also been measured. The proliferation of B cells stimulated by lipopolysaccharide declines with age but less strikingly than the decline in the proliferation of T cells stimulated by PHA (Gerbase-DeLima, WilKinson, Smith and Walford, 1974). However, in cases where the response to a B cell mitogen such as lipopolysaccharide is impaired, the cellular basis of the defect remains uncertain as T cells were not removed. This is because T cell preparations from old mice have increased suppressor activity. The removal of T cells is necessary to distinguish a disfunction of the B-lymphocytes from suppression of a B lymphocyte response.

Transfer studies have been particularly helpful in unravelling the nature of the immune deficiency associated with aging. Such studies can distinguish between host effects on immune function and defects within the immune system itself. Furthermore the capacity of thymocytes or thymic hormone to reverse age-associated immune defects can be investigated in transfer studies. In critical studies, lymphocytes from young or old animals were used to reconstitute young, thymectomized, lethally irradiated, syngeneic mice. The first transfer study performed nearly a decade ago showed that 90% of the age-associated defect in the PFC response to sheep erythrocytes was attributed to the lymphoid cells from aged animals and only 10% of these defects could be attributed to the environment of the old host (Makinodan and Adler, 1975). Subsequently it was shown that the preferential loss of high affinity and IgG antibody observed in old animals results from changes in the lymphoid system and can be transferred to young animals by lymphocytes from old mice (Goidl, Innes and Weksler, 1976). Transfer studies have also shown that suppressor activity increases with age. Thus, when old spleen cells are mixed with young spleen cells and transferred to recipients, the immune response of recipients of cells from both old and young mice is less than the response of recipients given cells from young mice. Spleen cells from 12,24 or 34 month old mice when given with spleen cells from 2 to 3 month old mice inhibited the response of recipients which received only spleen cells from 2 to 3 month old mice. Suppression induced by spleen cells from old mice did not preferentially affect high affinity or IgG PFC, indicating that increased suppressor activity contributes to but does not account for the immune deficiency of aging.

The contributions of thymic involution to the characteristic features of the age-associated decline in the anti-DNP PFC response has also been studied in transfer studies. Young recipients reconstitute with old spleen cells express the impairment in the high affinity and IgG PFC characteristic of old animals. This fact permitted studies which provided insight into the cellular basis of immune senescence. Thus, the high affinity and IgG antibody response of recipients of old spleen cells was reconstituted if young thymocytes were transferred to recipients at the same time as the old spleen cells (Goidl, Innes and Weksler, 1976). The important contribution of thymic involution to immune senescence was also supported by the observation that adult thymectomy accelerated the appearance of age-associated immune defects (Weksler, Innes and Goldstein, 1978). Furthermore, transfer of old spleen cells to young recipients possessing intact glands reversed the age-associated defect after residence of old spleen cells in the presence of a young thymus gland for a period of time. Thus, improved immunological function of recipients of spleen cells from aged animals depended on an 8 week period of residence in young lethally irradiated mice with thymus glands. No effect was seen in thymectomized recipients of old spleen cells. Finally, the age-associated defects of old spleen cells could be reversed by thymic hormone. Incubation of old spleen cells with thymic hormone in vitro prior to cell transfer augmented the capacity of recipient mice to produce a high affinity and IgG antibody response (Weksler, Innes and Goldstein, 1978).

In summary, two characteristic age-associated defects in immune function, the loss of high affinity and IgG antibody production, are reversed

in young recipients of old spleen cells by the transfer of young thymocytes with old spleen cells, by exposure of old spleen cells to the thymus
gland in young recipient animals or by the incubation of old spleen cells
with thymic hormone prior to transfer. These observations strongly support
the contribution of thymic involution to immune senescence. Furthermore,re
versing these age-associated immune defects with thymic hormone also offers
a potential therapeutic strategy for the immune deficiency of aging.

AGING AND THE REGULATION OF THE IMMUNE RESPONSE.

The involution of the thymus gland and the decline in the serum concen
tration of thymic hormone precede the loss of immune competence with age.
These events suggest that immune senescence might result from thymic deficiency state in man. However, deficiency of thymic function does not ade-
quately describe the complexity of immune senescence. In contranst to many
immune deficiency states, immune senescence is not associated with the loss
of a specific lymphocyte subpopulation or an immunoglobulin class. Furthermore, the pertubations of immune functions observed during immune senescence are more complex and varied than in most immunodeficiency states. The ran
ge of immunological pertubations e.g. autoantibody formation, increasing
difficulty of tolerance induction, monoclonal immunoglobulin production,are
not usually associated with immune deficiency. However, if the immune system is a network of interacting and countervailing elements, it remains
possible that thymic involution results not only in immune deficiency but
also in alteration in immune regulation.

It has been known for some years that the incidence of autoantibodies
in humans and experimental animals increases with age. Less than 5% of healthy humans under 40 years of age have autoantibodies to thyroglobulin,to
DNA or to immunoglobulin (rheumatoid factor). With age the frequency of the
se autoantibodies increases progressively so that 30 to 40 per cent of the
healthy individuals over 80 years of age have one or more of the autoantibodies (Hallgren, Buckley, Gilbertsen and Yunis, 1973). It is important to
note that elderly persons with these autoantibodies, do not have the clini

cal manifestations of autoimmune disease observed in young persons with the
se autoantibodies. This is not to say that these autoantibodies do not have
pathologic significance. An immunologic theory of aging (Walford, 1969)
restes on the thesis that autoimmune damage to cells and tissues plays an im
portant pathogenic mechanism in aging. Not only can autoantibodies directly
damage cells and tissues but the coexistence of autoantibodies and autoantigens can lead to the circulation of immune complexes. Recently it has
been found that nearly half the number of healthy persons over the age of
65 have high levels of circulating immune complexes (Day and Weksler,
1980). The pathogenic role of circulating immune complexes in vascular di
sease with in autoimmune disease is well known. Whether healthy older subjects with high levels of immune complexes are at greater risk of developing vascular or renal disease than are age matched subjects without circulating immune complexes is not known. This is a most important question
relating immune senescence to arterioscleroris, an important disease of
aging.

The presence of autoantibodies in elderly humans is not the only evidence of impaired regulating of B cell function. Altered B cell functions
is also manifested by the presence of benign monoclonal immunoglobulins.
The incidence of benign monoclonal gammapathy increases with age (Axels-
son, Bachmann and Hallen, 1966). These proteins are not associated with
the body lesions or malignant transformation of plasma cells seen in myeloma. Rather the increased frequency of these monoclonal proteins appear
to be yet another manifestation of impaired B cell regulation. Animals stu
dies have also shown that there is an increased frequency of benign monoclonal immunoglobulin with age and that the incidence of these monoclonal
proteins in old animals increase after thymectomy (Radl, DeGlopper, Van
den Berg and Van Zwieten, 1980). Thus, thymic involution may play an important role in the expression of age-associated benign monoclonal gamma
pathy.

The defense of the host against autoantibodies rests with immune mecha
nisms that mediate self tolerance. Two immune phenomena are though to

maintain self-tolerance and thereby prevent the appearance of auto-antibodies. Low levels of autologous antigens are believed to induce T-cell tolerance and activate suppressor T cells. As the activation of the autoreactive B cell depends upon helper T cell activity, T cell tolerance serves
as a primary defense mechanism against autoantibodies production. Suppres
sor T cells serve as a "back up" system to control the expression of autoreactive B cells activated by mechanisms which bypass the requirement for
T cell help. Both these mechanisms are affected by age. The impaired high
affinity antibody response seen in old animals probably reflects the loss
of B&T lymphocytes with high affinity receptors for antigen. If self-tolerance and the activation of T suppressor cells depends upon interaction
with low concentration of autologous antigens, the loss of high affinity
antigen receptors may impair these mechanisms. Thus, larger concentration
of autologous antigens may be required to activate low affinity T cells
than the amount of autologous antigens present in the circulation. Thus,
the maintainence of self-tolerance would be compromised with age.

Experimental evidence shows that tolerance is more difficult to induce
as animals grow old. This is true of both B and T-lymphocytes tolerance.
Administration of the B cell tolerogen, DNP-D-GL, prior to immunization
with DNP-BGG dramatically reduces the anti-DNP PFC response in young mice.
This method to induce B cell tolerance has been compared in mice of different ages (Dobken, Weksler and Siskin, 1980). The ease of tolerance induc
tion was quantitated by determining the dose of toleragen necessary to re
duce the anti-DNP PFC response by 50%. Very much greater amounts of tolerogen were required to induce this level of tolerance in old mice than in
young mice. The difficulty of inducing B cell tolerance in old mice was attributable to the lymphoid system and could not be related to change in to
lerogen processing or other host factors. The greater dose of tolerogen re
quired to induce B cell tolerance in old mice is compatible with the thesis
that B cells from old animals have lost receptors with high affinity for
the tolerogen.

Although there is less known about the affinity of the T cell antigen receptors, there is preliminary evidence that there is also a loss of T cells with high affinity receptors for antigen with age. Thus, the affini ty of cytotoxic T cells for target cells is lower in old as compared to young mice (Zharhardy and Gershon, 1980). T cell mediated carrier toleran ce has also been measured in animals of different ages. (DeKruyff, et al., 1980). The injection of untracentrifuged BGG prior to immunization with DNP-BGG results in a decrease in the anti-DNP PFC response. As was obser ved in B cells tolerance a higher dose of tolerogen was required in old mice to induce the same degree of tolerance achieved with a lower of to lerogen in young mice. Similary, transfer studies showed that the age-as sociated changes in the ease of T cell tolerance induction rested with two lymphocyte populations and not other factors.

Suppressor cells play an important role in the regulation of the immu ne response. While most attention has been devoted to T-lymphocytes with suppressor activity, there is evidence that non T-lymphocytes including mo nocytes and B-lymphocytes can also "down regulate" the immune response. Al tered suppressor cell activity has been documented in several diseases cha racterized by immune deficiency or autoimmunity. In general, high levels of suppressor activity have been associated with immune deficiency and low levels of suppressor activity with autoimmunity.

As the immune alterations associated with aging include both immune de ficiency to foreign antigens and autoimmunity, it has been suggested that different subpopulations of suppressor cells regulate immune responses to self and foreign antigens. There is considerable evidence that spontaneous suppressor activity for foreign antigens is increased in old humans and ex perimental animals. Thus, the human non-B-lymphocyte population (monocytes and/or T-lymphocytes) inhibit the in vitro synthesis of antibody by auto logous B cells. Spleen cells from old mice suppress the in vitro and in vi vo antibody response of syngeneic spleen cells. In animals where more pre cise assessment of the changing level of suppressor activity with age has been carried out, suppressor activity increases markedly after the mice re ach 12 months of age, one third their maximal lifespan. In contrast with the increase in spontaneous suppressor activity, non specific suppressor activity reamins constant or decreases with age (Hallgren and Yunis, 1977).

Lymphocytes exposed to lipopolysaccharide in vivo or in vitro are stimulated to produce autoantibodies. Lypopolysaccharide bypasses the requirement for T cell helper function and directly activates auto-reactive B cell. Lymphocytes from old animals are more susceptible to this effect. Thus, spleen cells from old mice incubated in vitro with lipopolysaccharide produce more autoantibody than do spleen cells from young mice (Meredith, Kristie and Walford, 1977). The increased expression of autoreactive B lymphocytes in old mice has been related to the age-associated loss of suppressor T cells which inhibit autoantibody production.

Autoantibodies, seen in old subjects reflect the disordered regulation of the immune response that accompanies aging. Certain autoantibodies react with regulatory T cells and thereby further the deregulation of the immune response. Thus, some elderly humans have an autoantibody with specificity for a population of suppressor T cells (Strelkauskas, 1980). These sub jects were found to have low levels of suppressor T cells suggesting that an autoantibody associated with aging might not only result from impaired suppressor activity but contribute to the deficiency of suppressor activity. A reverberating circuit would be developed which would thereby perpetuate the autoimmune state.

Another set of autoantibodies are now recognized to play an important role in the normal regulation of the immune response. Auto-anti-idiotypic antibodies react with antibodies produced during an immune response. The an ti-idiotypic antibodies are specific for the antigen combining site of the immunoglobulin molecule. Recently it has been found that this special group of autoantibodies, like autoantibodies in general, are produced in greater amount in old mice (Goidl, Thorbecke, Weksler and Siskind, 1980.). Auto-anti-idiotypic antibodies have the capacity to inhibit antibody secretion by interacting with the antibody producing B-lymphocyte. When the auto-anti-idiotypic antibodies, boung to the surface of lymphocytes from old mice, are removed, the impaired antibody response of lymphocytes from old mice is to a considerable extent reversed.

In summary, a complex set of immunoregulatory forces occur with aging, that can explain both the immunodeficiency and enhanced autoreactivity that occur in old humans and experimental animals. Resistance to tolerance induction and increased susceptibility to the activation of autoreactive B lymphocytes contribute to autoantibody formation. Increased suppressor cell activity and increased autoanti-idiotypic antibody appear to excessively "down regulate" the immune response and contribute to the immunodeficiency of aging.

BIOLOGICAL SIGNIFICANCE OF IMMUNE SENESCENCE

There are several lines of evidence that suggest that immune senescence may play an important role not only in the diseases which prevent animals from reaching the maximal lifespan of the species but in establishing the maximal lifespan of a species. The finding that genes of the major histocompatibility complex influence the rate of immune senescence as well as the maximal lifespan indicates the close relationship between the immune system and aging. Furthermore, two means to increase the maximal lifespan of animals, undernutrition and reduction in body temperature, are both associated with a prolongation of immunological vigor. There is a wide variation in immune competence among humans after middle age. Preliminary evidence points to an association between immune competence and long life span. Thus, old humans with autoantibodies (MacKay, 1972), with low suppressor activity (Hallgren and Yunis, 1980) or with gretly impaired cutaneous delayed by hypersensitivity (Robert-Thompson, Wittingham, Younchayud and MacKay, 1974) are at increased risk of death. Whether these relationships are casual i.e. poor immune function leads to shortened survival, requires additional, prospective studies.

Whether or not future work will sustain an immunologic theory of aging, it is almost certain that immune senescence plays an important part in the increased susceptibility of old humans to the diseases of aging. The increased incidence of infection clearly can be related to the loss of immune

184

competence. It is also likely that immune senescence contributes to the increased incidence of neoplastic disease among the elderly, either in its genesis or its progression. Finally, the disordered state of self tolerance, the formation of autoantibodies and the circulation of immune complex may accelerate arteriosclerotic vascular disease. The study of these interactions not only offer a better understanding of pathogenic mechanism of the disease of aging but may offer means to influence the development of these diseases by immune therapy.

References

Adler, W.H., Chrest, F.J., 1979. The mitogen response assay as a measure of immune deficiency of aging mice. In: Siskind, G.W., Litwin, S.D., Weksler, M.E., Developmental Immunology (Eds.), Grune and Stratton, New York, p. 233-246.

Axelsoon, U., Bachmann, R., Hallen, J., 1966. Frequency of pathological proteins (M-components) in 6, 995 sera from and adult population. Acta Med. Scand. 179-235-47.

Bach, J.F., Papiernik, M., Levasseur, P., Dardenne, M., Barois, A., Le Brigand, H., 1972. Evidence for a serum-factor secreted by the human thymus. Lancet 2:1056-1058.

Bierman, E.L., 1978. The effect of donor age on the in vitro life span of cultured human arterial smooth-muscle cells. In vitro 14 (11): 951-5.

Boyd, E., 1932. The weight of the thymus gland in health and in disease. Amer.J. Dis. Children 43:1162-1214.

Callard, R.E., Basten, A., Waters, L.K., 1977. Immune function in aged mice II B-cell function. Cell Immunol. 31:26-36.

Cutler, R.C., 1875. Evolution of human longevity and the genetic complexity governing aging rate. Proc. Natl. Acad. Sci. USA 72 (11): 4 664-8.

Day, N., Weksler, M.E., 1980. Unpublished observation.

DeKruyff, R.H., Rinnoy-Kan, E.A., Weksler, M.E., Siskind, G.W., Effect of aging on T-cell tolerance induction. Cell Immunol., in press.

DeKruyff, R.H., Kim, Y.T., Siskind, G.W., Weksler, M.E., 1980. Age related changes in the in vitro immune response: increased suppressor activity in immature aged mice. J. Immunol. (4): 125:142-147.

Dobken, J., Weksler, M.E., Siskind, G.W., 1980. Effect of age on ease of B-cell tolerance induction. Cell Immunol. 55:66-73.

Fernandez, A., MacSween, J., 1980. Decreased autologous mixed lymphocyte reaction with aging. Mech. Ageing. Dev. 12:245-248.

Garbase-DeLima, M.J., Wilkinson, J., Smith, G.S., Walford, R.L., 1974. Aged-related decline in thymic independent immune function in a long-lived mouse strain. J. Gerontology. 29:261-8.

Gillis, S., Kozak, R., Durante, M., Weksler, M.E., 1981. Immunological stu
  dies of aging. Decreased production of aged humans. J. Clin. Invest.
  67-931.
Goidl, E.A., Innes, J.B., Weksler, M.E., 1976. Immunological studies of
  aging II. Loss of IgG and high avidity plaque forming cells and increased suppressor cell activity in aging mice. J. Exp. Med., 144:
  1037-1048.
Goidl, E.A., Thombercke, G.J., Weksler, M.E. and Siskind, G.W., 1980. Production of auto-anti-idiotypic antibody during the normal immune response: change in the auto-anti-idiotypic response and the idiotypic
  repertoire associated with age. Proc. Nat. Acad. Sci. USA.
Goodwing, J.S. , Messner, R.P., 1979. Sensitivity of lymphocytes to prosta
  glandin E_2 increases in subjects over age 70. J. Clin. Invest. 64(2)
  434-9.
Gupta, S., Good, R.A., 1979. Subpopulation of human T-lymphocytes X altera
  tions in T, B, third population cells, and T- cells with receptors for
  T mu or T gamma immunoglabulin in aging humans. J. Immunol. 122 (4)
  1214-1219.
Hallgren, H.M., Yunis, E.J., 1980. In: Segre, D., Smith, L., (Eds) Immuno -
  logical aspects of aging, Marcel Dekker: N.Y.
Hallgren, H.M., Buckely, C.E., Gilbersten, V.A., Yunis, E.J., 1973. Lymphocyte phytohenmagglutinin responsivenness, immunoglobulins and auto-antibodies in aging humans. J. Immunol. 111. 1101-1107.
Hallgren, H.M., Yunis, E.J., 1977. Suppressor lymphocytes in young and a-
  ged humans. J. Immunol. 118: 2004-2008.
Hefton, J.M., Darlington, G., Casazza, B.A., Weksler, M.E., 1980. Immunolo
  gical studies of aging. V. Impaired proliferation of PHA responsiveness in human lymphocytes in culture. J. Immunol. 125: (2) 1007-1010.
Hirokawa, J., Makinodan, T., 1975. Thymic involution: effect in T-cell dif
  ferentiation . J. Immunol. 114 (6): 1659-64.
Inkeles, B., Innes, J.B., Kuntz, M.M., Kadish, A.S., Weksler, M.E., 1977.
  Immunological studies of aging III Cytokinetic basis for the impaired
  response of lymphocytes from aged humans to plant lectins. J. Exp. Med.
  145:1176-87.
Kim, Y.T., Siskind, G.W., Weksler, M.E., Cellular basis of the impaired im
  mune response of elderly humans. In: Fauci, A.S., Ballieux, R. (Eds.)
  Human B cell functions: activation and immunoregulation, Raven Press,
  in press.
Lewis, V.M., Twomey, J.J., Bealmear, P., Goldstein, G., Good , R.A., 1978.
  Age, thymic involution and circulating thymic hormones activity. J.
  Clin. Endo. Metabol. 47:145-150.
Mackay, I., 1972. Aging and Immunological function in man. Gerontologia
  18:825-304.
Makinodan, T., Adler, W.H., 1975. Effects of aging on the differentiation
  and proliferative potentials of cells of the immune system. Fed. Proc.
  32 (2): 152-8.
Martin, G.M., Spague, C.A., Epstein, C.J., 1970. Replicative life span of
  cultivated human cells: effects of donors' age, tissue and genotype.

Lab. Invest. 23:86-92

Meredith, P.J., Kristie, J.A., Walford, R.L., 1979. Aging increases expression of LPS induced autoantibody-secreting B cell. J. Immunol. 122:87.

Nilsson, B.S., 1971. In vitro lymphocyte reactivity to PPD and phytohemagglutin in relation to PPD skin reactivity and age. Scan J. Dis 52:39-47.

Paul, J.R., Brunnell, W.W., 1932. The presence of heterophile antibodies in infectious monocleosis. Am. J. Med. Sci. 183-90

Radl, J., DeGlopper, E., Vanderberg, P., Van Zwieten, M.J., 1980. Idiopathic paraproteimemia III. Increased frequency of paraproteimemia in thymectomized mice and in aging. J. Immunol. 125: 31-35.

Robert-Thompson, I.G., Wittingham, S., Youngchaiyud, U., Mackay, T.R., 1974. Aging immune response and mortality. Lancet. 2:368-70.

Rosenstein, M.M., Strausser, H.R., 1980. Macrophage-induced T-cell mitogen suppression with age. J. Retic. Endothel. Soc. 27: 159-166.

Singh, J., Singh, A.K., 1979. Age related changes in human thymus. Clin. Exp. Immunol. 37:507-511.

Singhal, S.K., Roder, J.C., Duwe, A.K., 1979. Suppressor cells in immunosenescence. Fed. Proc. 37 (5): 1245-52.

Smith, G.S., Walford, R.L., 1977. Influence of the main histocompatibility complex on aging in mice. Nature 270:727-729.

Strelkauskas, A., 1980. Autoantibodies to a regulatory T-cell subset in human aging. In: Segre, D., and Smith (eds.) Immunological Aspects of Aging. Marcel Dekker, N.Y., in press.

Stutman, O., 1972. Lymphocyte subpopulations in NZB mice: deficit of thymus-dependent lymphocytes. J. Immunol. 109:602-211.

Szewczuck, M.R., DeKruyff, R.H., Weksler, M.E., Siskind, G.W., Ontogeny of B lymphocyte function VIII. Failure of thymus cells from aged donors to induce the functional maturation of B lymphocytes from immature donors. Exp. J. Immunol. , in press.

Thomsen, O., Kettel, K., 1929. Die starke di menschlichen isoagglutine und entsprechenden blutkorperchenrezeptore in verschiedenen lebensaltein. Z. Immunoforsch. 63:67-93.

Walford, D.S., Wilkens, R.F., decker, J.L., 1968. Impaired delayed hypersensitivity in an aging population association with antinuclear reactivity and rheumatoid. JAMA 203:831-4; 831-834.

Walford, R.L., 1969. The immunologic theory of Aging. Munksguard. Copenhagen.

Weksler, M.E., Hutteroth, T.H., 1974. Impaired lymphocyte function in aged humans. J. Clin. Invest. 53:99-104.

Weksler, M.E., Innes, J.B., Goldstein, G., 1978. Immunological studies of aging IV. The contribution of thymic involution to the immune deficiencies of aging mice and reversal with thymopoietin. J. Exp. Med. 148: 996-1006.

Zharhary, D., Gershon, H., 1980. T-cytotoxic reactivity of senescent mice. In: Proceeding of Fourth International Congress of Immunology. Paris.

AUTOROSETTES AND AUTOLOGOUS MIXED LYMPHOCYTE REACTION IN HUMAN : TWO AGE-AND SEX-RELATED MODELS

Catherine Fournier, Han Ping Chen and Jeannine Charreire

INSERM U 25 - Hôpital Necker - 161, rue de Sèvres -

75015 Paris - France

ABSTRACT

Our studies on ageing were focused on two in vitro models of autologous responses of human peripheral blood lymphocytes. We investigated
first a T cell subset which binds autologous erythrocytes and forms spontaneous and stable autorosettes, and second, the proliferative response
of T cells towards autologous non-T cells. Both systems were shown to
be age and sex-related : indeed, women and mostly older ones, exhibited
significantly enhanced responses. The involvement of autorosette forming
cells (A-RFC) in the autologous proliferative response was strongly suggested by the fact that the removal of A-RFC abolished the autologous
cultures.

INTRODUCTION

The alteration of both humoral and cell-mediated immune functions
observed with ageing is presently well documented (for review see Yunis
et al., 1979). The impairment of T cell parameters is not surprising
since the senescence is associated with the involution of the thymus
gland. What is paradoxical is that this decline is often accompanied by
an increase in autoantibody production (Whitthingham et al., 1969 ; Shu
et al.,1975) and the appearance of autoimmune diseases (Good and Yunis,
1974). It is not clear whether this phenomenon reflects a rise of
"forbidden clones" which react against the host or an imbalance in T cell
subsets in the elderly which leads to a dysfunction of the suppressor
cell sets. It was our goal to examine the autologous reactions which
occur in every healthy subject and their behavior in age individuals.
For that purpose we have investigated in human peripheral blood lymphocytes (PBL) two models of autologous responses in vitro, in relationship
to the age the sex of the subjects.

MATERIALS AND METHODS

Isolation of mononuclear cells (MNC) and non-T cells

Human blood from healthy donors was diluted 1/3 in Hanks' balanced salt solution (HBSS) supplemented with 1% antibiotics (Penicillin, Streptomycin, Flow) and centrifuged at 320g for 15 min on a mixture of Ficoll (Pharmacia) and Telebrix 38 (sodium ioxitalamate and meglumin ioxitalamate, Guerbet, France). The cells at the interface were collected, pooled, and washed twice in HBSS. Non-T cells were separated by layering E rosette suspensions performed as previously described (Fournier and Charreire, 1977) on a Ficoll-Telebrix mixture. After centrifugation at 280 g for 20 min at room temperature, the depleted cells at the interface were collected, pooled and washed in HBSS.

Formation and depletion of autorosette-forming cells (A-RFC)

Autorosettes were performed by centrifugation at 150 g for 5 min of 1.5×10^6 MNC mixed with various amounts of washed autologous erythrocytes in a total volume of 0.25 ml. After overnight incubation at 4°C, A-RFC were counted and the results expressed per 1000 lymphocytes. Several ratios of autologous red blood cells to white cells (A-RBC/WC) ranging from 4/1 to 128/1 were tested. Removal of A-RFC was performed after the incubation at 4°C by centrifugation of autorosette suspension on a Ficoll-Telebrix mixture, as described above.

Culture conditions

All cell suspensions (3×10^6/ml) were prepared in RPMI 1640 (supplemented with 2 mM glutamine, 1% antibiotics (Flow) and 20% heat-inactivated autologous plasma. Autologous and allogeneic MLR were conducted in quadruplicate in round-bottomed microplates by mixing 0.1 ml of unfractionated MNC with an equal volume of irradiated (2000 R) autologous non-T cells or allogeneic MNC. After a 5-day incubation at 37°C in 5% CO_2 in humidified air, the cultures were pulsed with 1 μCi of ^{3}H thymidine and 20 hours later the cells were harvested and their radioactivity was determined by liquid scintillation counting. In some experiments testosterone or estradiol (Sigma) were added at final concentrations of 10^{-7}, 10^{-9} and 10^{-11} M in the cultures at day 0.

189

RESULTS

1. Autologous erythrocyte binding cells

    For the last three years, we have been engaged in the study of the existence of lymphocytes which bind autologous erythrocytes to form rosettes. Using a technique that detects spontaneous and stable auto-rosette forming cells (A-RFC) we have characterized a T cell subset found with high incidence in the thymus (25-30%) but low levels in the periphery (Fournier and Charreire, 1978). However, as shown in Fig.1, the autorosette percentages increased with the age of the subjects. This observation was consistent irrespective of the erythrocyte to lymphocyte ratio used for autorosette formation. Interestingly, the two female groups over 50 years old displayed significantly higher numbers of A-RFC (at high A-RBC/WC ratios) than did the corresponding aged males. Thus, the A-RFC represent a small proportion of T cells which augments with age, mostly in the female's peripheral blood.

FIGURE 1 – Autorosette levels at different ratios of autologous
red blood cells to white cells (A-RBC/WC) in relationship
to age and sex.

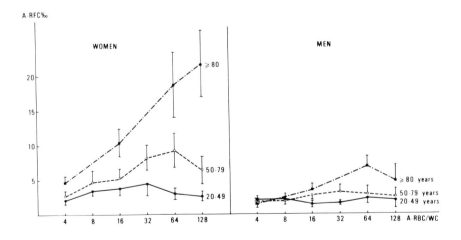

2. Autologous proliferative response

Lymphocytes from healthy donors can be stimulated in vitro by irradiated autologous non T cells, giving rise to a proliferative response (Opelz et al.,1975 and Kuntz et al.,1976). Using unfractionated MNC as responder cells and irradiated autologous E rosette-depleted cells as stimulators, we have analyzed the proliferative response of normal individuals in relation to their age and sex. In the two age groups considered, we have shown that female subjects displayed enhanced responses compared with that of males. The difference was very significant ($p < 0.02$) in the older group (Fig.2). Moreover, the responses of women over 50 years old were significantly increased in

FIGURE 2 - Autologous mixed lymphocyte reaction in relationship to age and sex

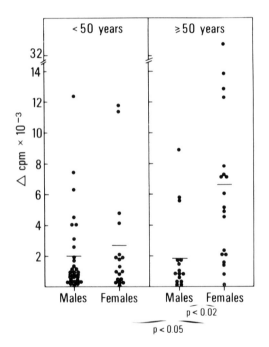

comparison with the younger female group ($p < 0.05$). In contrast, the response to allogeneic cells of the same donors were not modified (Fig.3).

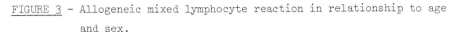

FIGURE 3 - Allogeneic mixed lymphocyte reaction in relationship to age
and sex.

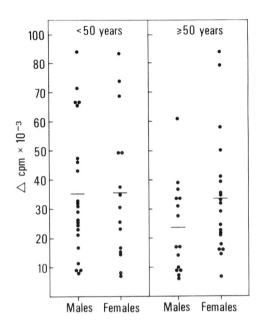

The fact that we have used 20% autologous plasma in the culture medium in order to avoid any stimulation by allogeneic or xenogeneic serum
raised two questions : 1/ does the plasma of older individuals contain
autoantibodies which could stimulate the autologous response ? and
2/ since females showed higher responses than males, is there any influence of sex hormones in our system ?

In order to resolve these problems, we have tested the autologous
proliferative responses of lymphocytes either in autologous plasma or
in a pool of AB serum. As shown in Fig.4, in 9 out of 10 experiments the
level of stimulation was identical, irrespective of the origin of the
serum used. A higher response in AB serum was only observed in one case
and finally the mean values of stimulation obtained in the presence of
autologous plasma were very similar to those with AB serum (Fig.4).

The eventual influence of sex hormones was evaluated by adding either
testosterone or estradiol to the cultures. In 10 experiments (5 males
and 5 females) the presence of those hormones during the culture did not
modify the thymidine incorporation obtained in autologous or allogeneic

cultures (Table 1). Thus, it appears that the use of autologous plasma
is not responsible for an enhanced autologous response in the elderly.

FIGURE 4 - Influence of autologous plasma versus allogeneic AB serum in
the autologous mixed lymphocyte reaction (A-MLR)
•—• individual responses : o--o mean values

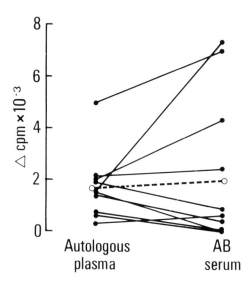

TABLE 1 - Autologous and allogeneic MLR of lymphocytes from males and females in the presence of sex hormones (Testosterone or Estradiol)
at different concentrations. The results are expressed as means
± S.E.M.of stimulation indexes (cpm of stimulated culture divided by cpm of responding lymphocytes alone incubated in the
presence of the same hormone concentration).

Hormone concentration		MALES (n = 5)		FEMALES (n = 5)	
		Autologous MLR	Allogeneic MLR	Autologous MLR	Allogeneic MLR
0		3.3 + 1.4	20.5 + 5.3	3.0 + 1.2	17.8 + 5.5
Testosterone	10^{-11}M	3.7 + 1.4	22.8 + 5.4	3.0 + 0.6	14.4 ± 5.3
	10^{-9}M	3.8 + 1.4	21.0 + 4,4	2.9 + 1.8	14.9 ± 4.5
	10^{-7}M	3.2 + 1.4	23.1 + 5.9	3.0 + 1.6	15.4 ± 4.5
Estradiol	10^{-11}M	3.1 + 1.6	20.5 + 5.5	2.5 + 1.5	13.3 + 3.8
	10^{-9}M	3.2 + 0.9	19.1 + 4.3	2.1 + 1.1	12.0 + 3.2
	10^{-7}M	3.0 + 1.4	18.0 + 4.1	2.0 + 1.0	11.6 ± 2.3

DISCUSSION

This study extends our understanding on autoreactivity of normal
individuals and further provides evidence that the autologous reactions
are age and sex-dependent. Using autorosette formation, we were able to
detect a small subset of lymphocytes which are involved in the recognition
of autologous erythrocytes. We have previously developed a series of arguments which attest that the A-RFC belong to the T cell lineage (Fournier
and Charreire, 1977, 1978 and 1980). In this respect, our findings are
in agreement with others (for review see Gallinger et al.,1980). What is
more controversial is the level of this subpopulation in peripheral blood.
In the paper of Gallinger et al. cited above, it appears that our percentages are the lowest reported in the literature. There is actually no doubt
that this wide range of results obtained in different laboratories depends
upon the techniques used. In our assay we detect only the cells which bind
autologous erythrocytes with high avidity. More precisely, we mix lymphocytes and erythrocytes without any previous enzyme treatment, in serum
free medium, and for the resuspension of the rosettes we use a highly
reproducible procedure on a rotating platform. Interestingly, it is under
these technical conditions that we find an increase in A-RFC associated
with ageing and mostly for the females. Indeed, such an age and sex dependency of autorosettes could not be found by those who reported high levels
of A-RFC. Moreover, from a theoretical point of view, our low numbers of
circulating A-RFC are fully compatible with the existence of an "autoreactive" T cell subpopulation in peripheral blood. In addition, as we
reported elsewhere (Fournier and Charreire, 1981), the impairment of
autologous mixed lymphocyte reaction (A-MLR) after removal of the high
avidity autorosettes, strongly suggests that this small subset of T cells
belongs to the responder cells of A-MLR. Similar conclusions have been
reached by others (Palacios et al.,1980 and Tomonari et al., 1980). Our
hypothesis is further supported by the finding that the response in A-MLR
is age and sex-related : the proliferative response in older subjects is
higher than that in younger ones and this increase is more pronounced for
women. As in autorosette formation, the rise in response appears from the
age of 50 years, indicating that the same T cell subset is involved in
both tests.

In conclusion, our data demonstrate the existence in the peripheral blood of healthy individuals of cells which are involved in self-reactivity in vitro. These potentially autoreactive cells are increased in senescence and are found with higher incidence in female subjects. Whether these cells could account for the age-associated increase in frequency of autoimmune disorders in older females remains to be resolved.

ACKNOWLEDGMENTS

The authors are indebted to Mrs. S.MISTOU for her excellent technical assistance and to Miss J.JACOBSON for her editorial assistance.

REFERENCES

Fournier,C. and Charreire,J. : Increase in autologous erythrocyte binding by T cells with ageing in man. Clin.exp.Immunol., 29 : 468-473,1977.

Fournier,C. and Charreire, J.: Activation of a human T cell subpopulation bearing receptors for autologous erythrocytes by concanavalin A. J.Immunol., 121 :771-776, 1978.

Fournier,C. and Charreire,J.: Autoreactivity of human peripheral blood lymphocytes : relationship between autorosettes and autologous proliferative response. in "New Trends in Human Immunology and Cancer Immunotherapy" Ed. B.Serrou and C.Rosenfeld : pp 97-106 (Doin, Paris 1980).

Fournier,C. and Charreire,J. : Autologous mixed lymphocyte reaction in man. I. Relationship with age and sex. Cell.Immunol. in press ,1981.

Gallinger,L.A., Pross,H.F. and Baines,M.G. :Human lymphocyte/human erythrocyte rosettes. I. Blood "H" rosettes are high affinity E rosette-forming T lymphocytes occuring in high frequency. Int.J.Cancer, 26 : 139-150, 1980.

Good,R.A. and Yunis,E.J. : Association of autoimmunity, immunodeficiency and aging in man, rabbits and mice. Fed.Proc. 33 : 2040-2050, 1974.

Kuntz,M.M., Innes,J.B. and Weksler,M.E. : Lymphocyte transformation induced by autologous cells. IV. Human T lymphocyte proliferation induced by autologous or allogeneic non-T lymphocytes. J.exp.Med. 143 : 1042-1054, 1976.

Opelz,G., Kichi,M., Takasugi,M. and Terasaki,P.I.: Autologous stimulation of human lymphocyte subpopulations. J.exp.Med. 142 : 1327-1333, 1975.

Palacios,R., Llorente,L., Alarcon-Segovia,D., Ruiz-Arguelles,A. and Diaz-Jouanen,E.: Autologous rosette forming T cells as the responding cells in human autologous mixed lymphocyte reaction. J.Clin.Invest. 65 : 1527-1530, 1980.

Shu,S., Nigengard,R.J., Hale,W.L. and Beutner,E.H.: Incidence and titers of antinuclear, antismooth muscle and other autoantibodies in blood donors. J.Lab.Clin.Med. 86 : 259-265, 1975.

Tomonari,K., Wakisaka,A. and Aizawa,M.: Self recognition by autologous mixed lymphocyte reaction-primed cells. J.Immunol. 125 : 1596-1600, 1980.

Whitthingham,S., Irwin,J., Mackay,I.R., Marsh,S. and Cowling,D.C. : Autoantibodies in healthy subjects. Aust.Ann.Med. 18 :130-134, 1969.

Yunis,E.J., Handwerger,B.S., Hallgren,H.M., Good,R.A. and Fernandes,G. : Aging and immunity. in " Mechanisms of Immunopathology" Ed.S.Cohen, P.A.Ward and R.T. Mc Cluskey, pp 91-106 (J.Wiley, New York, 1979).

SELECTIVE DEFICIENCY OF T-LYMPHOCYTE SUBSET(S) IN AGED AND IN DOWN'S SYNDROME SUBJECTS

C. Franceschi, F. Licastro, M. Chiricolo, M. Zannotti, N. Fabris,
E. Mocchegiani, L. Tabacchi, F. Barboni and M. Masi

Institute of General Pathology, Institute of General Histology and Embrio
logy and Department of Pediatrics, University of Bologna, Experimental Ge
rontology Center I.N.R.C.A., Research Department, Ancona, and Laboratory
of Clinical Analysis of "M. Malpighi" Hospital, Bologna - Italy

ABSTRACT

The immunocompetence of 22 aged subjects ($90+1$ yr old) and of 15 su
bjects with Down's syndrome (DS) was studied and compared with 21 young
subjects and 14 subjects with normal karyotype, respectively. A marked
decrease in PHA response and autologous mixed lymphocyte reaction (MLR)
of T enriched lymphocytes from both old and DS subjects was observed.The
responsiveness of T enriched lymphocytes to allogeneic irradiated non-T
cells was well preserved in both groups. The data suggest that an altera
tion of a subset(s) of T lymphocyte(s) with regulatory function and of
self-recognition is present in aged humans and DS patients.

INTRODUCTION

Aging is characterized by increased incidence of autoimmunity (Hall
gren et al., 1973) and neoplasia (Doll et al., 1970). Immunocompetence
progressively declines with age and according to many Authors an alteration of the T-cell compartment and particularly of T lymphocytes with
regulatory functions could account for the majority of the immunological
defects found in aged subjects (Makinodan and Kay, 1980). T lymphocyte
defects similar to those found in advanced age have been described in
DS (trisomy-21 or mongolism) (Franceschi et al., 1978). DS, i.e. the
most common human autosomal aberration, is characterized by a precocious
aging of the immune system (Bonetti et al., 1980) and is considered to
be the most representative "progeroid syndrome" among all human genetic
disorders (Martin, 1979).

Since autologous MLR is known to be a test for a subset of T lympho
cytes with regulatory function and has been found defective in humans
affected by autoimmune diseases (Sakane et al., 1978) and in autoimmune
prone mice (Smith and Pasternak, 1978) we have thought it worthwhile to
study autologous MLR in aged humans and in DS subjects.

To further investigate the basis of the T-cell defect in these two
groups we also measured the ability of enriched T lymphocytes to respond

in the presence of two other T-cell stimulants, such as phytohaemagglutinin (PHA) and allogeneic antigens in one-way MLR.

MATERIALS AND METHODS

22 subjects (5 males and 17 females) aged between 85 to 104 yr (mean
90+1 yr) were studied. 21 students and laboratory personnel (10 males
and 11 females) aged between 19 to 37 yr (mean 30+1 yr) comprised our
control group of young people.

Peripheral blood was also obtained from 15 DS subjects aged from 6
to 23 yr and from healthy sex- and aged-matched normal controls (10 to
27 yr). Both groups included noninstitutionalized subjects. The karyotype of all DS subjects had been examined and all had a nontranslocated
trysomy-21. All the subjects studied were apparently in good health.
Peripheral blood lymphocytes (PBL). PBL were separated by density gradient centrifugation through Ficoll-Hypaque (Böyum, 1968).
Peripheral blood T and B lymphocytes. Peripheral T lymphocytes were evaluated as E rosette forming cells (E-RFC) with sheep red blood cells
(SRBC) and B lymphocytes were detected using a polivalent fluorescein-co
njugated sheep antiserum to human heavy chains (Wellcome, England) as
described elsewhere (Franceschi et al., 1978).
T and non-T lymphocyte purification. Enriched T and non-T cells were
obtained by a rosetting technique using AET- (Pellegrino et al., 1975)
or neuraminidase- (Falasca et al., 1980) treated SRBC.
Autologous and allogeneic MLR and PHA stimulation. All these tests were
performed as described in details elsewhere (Franceschi et al., in press).

RESULTS

No difference was found between old and young subjects, as far as
peripheral blood leukocytes, lymphocytes and T and B lymphocytes are
concerned (data not shown). On the contrary T enriched lymphocyte respon
siveness to PHA of old and DS, subjects was markedly decreased.

TABLE 1 - PHA STIMULATION OF T ENRICHED LYMPHOCYTES FROM OLD AND DS
SUBJECTS AND THEIR CONTROLS

Subjects	without PHA	with PHA
Young (21)[a]	1 178 + 328[b]	79 032 + 9 480
Old (22)	1 366 + 595	40 753 + 4 013
P[c]	NS[d]	< 0.001
Normal (14)	1 082 + 239	98 975 + 8 274
Down (15)	846 + 491	61 519 + 4 932
P	NS	< 0.001

[a]Number of subjects studied; [b]the data are expressed as mean+SEM of
cpm; [c]statistical analysis was performed by Student's t test; [d]NS=
= not significant.

The responsiveness in autologous MLR was significantly decreased in both old and DS subjects in comparison with their control groups as shown in Table 2.

TABLE 2 - AUTOLOGOUS MLR IN OLD SUBJECTS, DS SUBJECTS AND THEIR CONTROLS

Subjects		Autologous MLR[a] (T cells + irradiated non-T cells)	P[b]
Young	(19)[c]	100	< 0.02
Old	(21)	46	
Normal	(13)	100	< 0.02
Down	(14)	53	

[a]Data are expressed as percentage of ^{3}H-thymidine incorporation in comparison with control groups = 100%; [b]significance according to the Student's t test; [c]number of subjects studied.

The responsiveness to allogeneic antigens (Table 3) was normal in DS subjects and slightly decreased in olde subjects.

TABLE 3 - ALLOGENEIC MLR IN OLD SUBJECTS, TRIS-21 SUBJECTS AND THEIR CONTROLS

Responder cells (T lymphocytes)	Stimulator cells (irradiated non-T cells)		P[a]
	Young	Old	
Young	100[b] (15)[c]	107 (12)	NS
Old	76 (18)	81 (18)	NS
P	NS	NS	
	Normal	Down	
Normal	100[b] (5)	124 (7)	NS
Down	101 (11)	106 (7)	NS
P	NS	NS	

[a]Significance according to the Student's t test; NS = not significant; [b]data are expressed as percentage of ^{3}H-thymidine incorporation in comparison to control groups = 100%; [c]number of combination performed.

CONCLUSIONS

The data presented show that T lymphocytes from both old and DS subjects are functionally impaired when stimulated with PHA and autologous antigens. On the contrary their responsiveness in presence of allo-geneic antigens is well preserved. Since it is known (Ilfeld et al., 1977) that T lymphocytes responding in autologous and allogeneic MLR be-long to different subsets, these data suggest the presence of a selecti-ve impairment of a T lymphocyte subpopulation in both these conditions.

Furthermore our data confirm and extend previous observations about the precocious aging of the immune system in DS subjects.

Although the biological significance of autologous MLR is not esta-blished a general agreement exists that such a reaction is related to an immune mechanism involved in self recognition as well as to the T cell regulatory function. An alteration of such mechanisms could explain many immune defects observed in aged humans and DS subjects and it could be related to the high incidence of autoimmunity and neoplasia observed in aging and DS.

This work was supported by Grant 80 01552.96 from the Italian Natio nal Research Council (C.N.R.) to C. Franceschi within the "Progetto Fi-nalizzato sul Controllo della Crescita Neoplastica - Sottoprogetto Con-trollo Immunitario" and by the Pallotti's Legacy for cancer research.

REFERENCES

Bonetti, F., Licastro, F., Chiricolo, M. and Franceschi, C., 1980. La sindrome di Down. Un invecchiamento precoce del sistema immunitario. Rec. Progr. in Med., 69: 679-709.

Böyum, A., 1968. Separation of leukocytes from blood and bone marrow. Scand. J. Clin. Lab. Invest., 21 (suppl. 97): 77-81.

Doll, R., Muir, C. and Waterhouse, J. (Editors), 1970. Cancer incidence in five Continents, U.I.C.C., Geneva.

Falasca, A., Franceschi, C., Rossi, C.A. and Stirpe, F., 1980. Mitogenic and haemagglutinating properties of a lectin purified from Hura crepitans seeds. Biochim. Biophys. Acta, 632: 95-105.

Franceschi, C., Licastro, F., Paolucci, P., Masi, M., Cavicchi, S. and Zannotti, M., 1978. T and B lymphocyte subpopulations in Down's syndrome. A study on not-institutionalized subjects. J. Ment. Defic. Res., 22: 179-191.

Franceschi, C., Licastro, F., Chiricolo, M., Bonetti, F., Zannotti, M., Fabris, N., Mocchegiani, E., Fantini, M.P., Paolucci, P. and Masi, M. Deficiency of autologous mixed lymphocyte reactions and serum thymic factor level in Down's syndrome. J. Immunol., (in press).

Hallgren, H.M., Buckley, C.E., Gilbertsen, V.A. and Yunis, E.J., 1973. Lymphocyte phytohemagglutinin responsiveness, immunoglobulins and autoantibodies in aging humans. J. Immunol. 111: 1101-1107.

Ilfeld, D.N., Krakauer, R.S. and Blease, R.M., 1977. Suppression of the human autologous mixed lymphocyte reactions by physiologic concen-trations of hydrocortisone. J. Immunol., 119: 428-431.

Makinodan, T. and Kay, M.B., 1980. Age influence on the immune system. Adv. Immunol., 29: 287-330.

Martin, G.M., 1979. Genetic and evolutionary aspects of aging. Fed. Proc. 38: 1962-1967.

Pellegrino, M.A., Ferrone, S., Dierich, M.P. and Reisfeld, R.A., 1975. Enhancement of sheep red blood cell human lymphocyte rosette formation by the sulphydryl compound 2-amino ethylisothiouronium bromide. Clin. Immunol. Immunopathol., 3: 324-333.

Sakane, T., Steinberg, A.D. and Green, I., 1978. Failure of autologous mixed lymphocyte reactions between T and non-T cells in patients with systemic lupus erythematosus. Proc. Natl. Acad. Sci., 75: 3464--3468.

Smith, J.B. and Pasternak,R.D.,1978. Syngeneic mixed lymphocyte reaction in mice: strain distribution, kinetics, partecipating cells and absence in NZB mice. J. Immunol., 121: 1889-1892.

BENIGN AND MALIGNANT MONOCLONAL GAMMOPATHY:
DIFFERENTIATION BY MEANS OF THE J CHAIN

E.J.E.G. Bast, B. van Camp[*] and R.E. Ballieux
Clinical Immunology Department, University
Hospital, Utrecht, The Netherlands and
*Clinical Haematology Department, Hospital
of the Free University (VUB), Brussels, Belgium.

ABSTRACT

A new technique is described facilitating the differential diagnosis between benign (BMG) and malignant IgG-type monoclonal gammopathy (MMG). Junction (J) chain was found in most of the malignant plasmacells and absent in most of cases of BMG. Using anti-idiotypic antisera instead of anti IgG, we found similar results. In one case malignancy was indicated by the presence of a high percentage J containing IgG plasmacells prior to clinical expression of multiple myeloma.

INTRODUCTION

Monoclonal gammopathy is defined by the presence of a homogeneous immunoglobulin (Ig) fraction in the serum. It is a rather frequent occurring phenomenon, especially in the aged. Only a minor proportion of these cases the M component can be ascribed to a underlying B cell malignancy (e.g. multiple myeloma). The majority represent the benign form, in which therapeutic intervention should be avoided. Differential diagnosis is important therefore, but has been hampered by the lack of unambiguous criteria, the only being clinical "presence or absence of progression" (Waldenström, 1974).

J chain, a polypeptide from polymeric Ig's (IgA and IgM) has been found also in immature IgG synthesizing cells both in vitro (Mestecky et al., 1977) and in vivo (Brandtzaeg, 1976). Since malignant cells may express more immature characteristics, we looked for the presence of J chain in cells of MMG and BMG, anticipating its presence in the first and absence in the latter case. We found this expected differential expression of J chain in 85% of the cases studied, thus allowing for a more solid diagnosis in this situation.

MATERIALS AND METHODS

We studied bone marrow samples from 91 patients (35 with MMG and 56 with BMG) and 17 controls. Cytocentrifuged cells were incubated sequentially with TRITC conjugated rabbit anti human J chain (RAHu/J-TRITC) provided by Dr. J. Mestecky (Mestecky et al., 1977) and FITC conjugated anti human IgG (Nordic, Tilburg, The Netherlands). In cases indicated specific anti-idiotypic antisera (made as described by Radl et al., 1978) anti IgD, anti κ or anti λ (Nordic), all conjugated with FITC, were used instead.

RESULTS

We found a significant differential expression of J chain in plasmacells from patients with MMG ($65 \pm 36\%$) versus BMG ($15 \pm 26\%$) and controls ($15 \pm 10\%$). Most of the patients in the MMG group (27 out of 35) expressed J chain in more than 50% of their IgG plasmacells, whereas in 48 out of 56 cases of BMG and all of the 17 controls this percentage was less than 35%. Whereas the difference between the groups was highly significant, the predictive value in individual patients is not absolute. In some MMG patients we did not find high percentages J chain containing IgG plasmacells, and in some patients, classified as having BMG we did find a high J content. Importantly, however, one of these cases proved to evolve a malignancy at later stage. In order to define the monoclonal plasma cell population more precisely we performed comparative staining experiments using patient's specific anti-idiotypic and anti IgG conjugates. In cases of both MMG and BMG the results are confluent (Fig. 2).

CONCLUSIONS

The presence or absence of J chain in plasmacells is an additional criterion in the differential diagnosis between IgG type MMG and BMG. This may relate the stage of maturity of the plasmacells; also physiologically immature IgG plasmacells are J chain positive, whereas this polypeptide from polymeric Ig is not detectable in mature IgG plasmacells. The sensitivity and the specificity of the method was 77% and 87% in a study on 91 patients. J chain may provide an early means of diagnosis; in one case of BMG, having a high percentage J chain containing plasmacells, MMG evolved lateron.

202

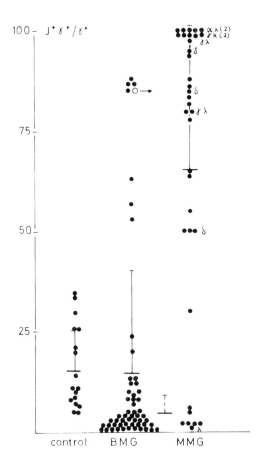

Fig. 1 J chain in IgG plasmacells
  Bone marrow slides from 35 patients with malignant monoclonal gammopathy (MMG), 56 with benign monoclonal gammopathy (BMG) and 17 controls
were sequentially incubated with anti-IgG FITC and anti-J chain TRITC.
In some exceptions other conjugates were used: λ, $\alpha\lambda$, $\gamma\lambda$: in bone
marrow from these patients a large number of the plasmacells were posi-
tive only for the λ chain and not for the H (α or γ) chain. These slides were stained with anti-λ FITC instead of anti-IgG FITC.$\gamma\kappa$: Slides
from these patients (having cells positive for only the κ chain but also
a large amount of cells positive for the whole IgGκ molecule) were
stained using anti-κ FITC instead of anti-IgG FITC. δ: These slides (IgD
myeloma) were stained using anti-IgD FITC instead of anti-IgG FITC. o→ :
This patient had a 5-year stable M component at the time of the bone
marrow sampling. Later he developed MMG.
  A significant difference was found in the MMG vs. BMG and the controls (P<0.0001).

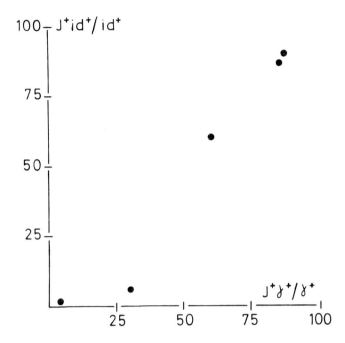

Fig. 2 Comparison of the percentages of J chain-positive cells within IgG or idiotype-positive cells in bone marrow smears from five patients. The percentages of J chain-positive cells within the IgG-containing cell population ($J^+\gamma^+/\gamma^+$) were significantly similar (r=0.97535, P<0.005) to the percentages of J chain-containing cells within the idiotype-positive cell population (J^+id^+/id^+).

REFERENCES

Brandtzaeg, P. (1976) Studies on J chain and binding site for secretory component in circulating B cells. II. The cytoplasm. Clin. Exp. Immunol. 25, 59.

Mestecky, J., Winchester, R.J., Hoffman, T. and Kunkel, H.S. (1977) Parallel synthesis of immunoglobulins and J-chain in pokeweed mitogen-stimulated normal cells and in lymphoblastoid cell lines. J. Exp. Med. 145, 760.

Radl, J., Glopper, E. and De Groot, G. (1978) Rapid, simple and reliable technique for preparation of antisera against idiotypes of homogeneous immunoglobulins. Vox Sang. 35, 10.

Waldenström, J.G. (1974) Benign monoclonal gammopathies. In: Multiple Myeloma and Related Disorders (ed. by M. Azar and M. Potter), Vol.I p. 247. Harper & Row, Hagerstown.

CSF OLIGOCLONAL PATTERN IN TWO CASES OF CEREBRAL AMYLOID ANGIOPATHY

E.Schuller[*], R.Escourolle[**], F. Gray[**],
H.Sagar[*], J.J.Hauw[**] .

[*]Laboratory of Neuro-Immunology and [**]Laboratory
of Neuropathology, Hôpital de la Salpêtrière
75651 Paris Cedex 13

ABSTRACT

CSF oligoclonal pattern of gamma zone is thought to be the expression of IgG local synthesis. This characteristic pattern was observed in the CSF of two aged (61 and 73 years old) male patients with progressive amnesia, disturbances of vigilancy, and impairment of psychological performances. Post-mortem pathological examination showed typical changes of amyloid angiopathy. Thus, the local synthesis of IgG might account for the amyloid deposits : these two observations suggest a new immunopathological mechanism of brain ageing.

INTRODUCTION

The pathophysiology of cerebral amyloid deposit in senile plaques and amyloid angiopathy is still obscure. A better knowledge of the mechanism of these changes would be of special interest for the following reasons :
1) They are characteristic of senile dementia of the Alzheimer type and/or of Alzheimer's disease (Escourolle and Poirier, 1976). These disorders of unknown etiology account for a large number of dementias in patients over age 55. In addition, senile plaques have been observed in other diseases, such as adult Down's syndrome. In the same way, amyloid angiopathy may be responsible for cerebral hemorrhages (Gudmunson,et al, 1972, Jellinger, 1977, Lee and Stemmermann, 1978) and perhaps, for some special forms of late-onset dementias (Okasaki, et al, 1979). Furthermore, senile plaques have been repeatedly reported in area H2 of the hippocampus of elderly apparently normal

people. Amyloid deposit in the brain has also been detected
in morphologically different plaques (amyloid plaques) of
mice inoculated with scrapie and of human kuru and
Creuzfeldt-Jakob disease, the transmissible nature of which
has been prooved.

2) The characteristic histochemical and ultrastructural
features of amyloid depend on the conformation of the
plaque-forming fibrils, i.e.twisted β-pleated sheets. This
structure may be related to different chemical compositions
(Glenner, 1978, Linke, 1978) "Primary" type of amyloid
fibril proteins found in acquired systemic amyloidoses
has been identified as the whole or part of immunoglobulin
light polypeptide chain (Lλ and Lk).
Amyloid deposits in "secondary" types of amyloidosis have
revealed the presence of a unique protein (protein AA).
Other types of amyloid protein, such as found in medullary
carcinome of the thyroid, primary hereditary amyloidosis
(Portuguese type) or senile cardiac amyloid for example,
have been described. (Linke, 1978). The chemical nature of
cerebral amyloid (S) is not known. As far as polarization
microscopic-histochemical studies are concerned, some senile
plaques behave as primary and some as secondary amyloid
(Kattenkamp and Stiller, 1973). The protein composition
of amyloid angiopathy is different (Powers and Spicer,
1977). Normal serum immunoglobulins diffuse into the
neuropil with a decreasing concentration gradient (Ishii
et al, 1975) We report here the unusual finding of oligoclonal features of CSF immunoglobulins in two patients with
pathologically proved cerebral amyloid changes.

PATIENTS AND METHODS

Case 1. The onset of troubles in this 61 year old male
patient was marked by progressive memory loss, impairment
of psychological performances and disturbances of level of
conciousness. Physical examination showed a mild defect of
cognitive functions, without focal neurological signs.
Blood pressure was normal. EEG showed diffuse slowing. The

patient's condition gradually deteriorated with exacerba-
tions and resolutions of his symptoms. He died at 64. Post-
mortem examination of the brain (1260 g) disclosed numerous
diffuse neuritic plaques and neurofibrillary tangles. The
senile changes were associated with vascular lesions :
focal ischemia often predominant in watershed areas with
small hemorrhages of various ages. The most striking changes identifies were the presence of numerous and widespread
lesions of amyloid angiopathy of both the congophilic and
dyshoric varieties.

Case 2. The onset of troubles in this 72 year old alcoholic
male patient living alone was thought to be sudden. He presented with a regressive coma followed by apathy. Examination after an acute confusional episode showed loss of memory, deterioration of intellectual functionning and disturbances of level of conciousness, with hypersomnia. Plan-
tar reflexes were in extension. Blood pressure was slightly
elevated (from 130/70 to 180/100 mm Hg ; mean value : 160-
95). EEG showed diffuse slowing. The patient died at 74
after gradual deterioration. Post mortem examination of the
brain (1170 g) showed small disseminated infarcts of the
basal ganglia, small hemorrhages in the left insula and a
few senile plaques and tangles in occipital, temporal and
frontal lobes. Amyloid angiopathy, essentially of the
dyshoric type, was seen in every examined area of cerebral
cortex.

CSF Analysis. Total protein was determinated by Lowry method using bovine serum albumin as standard. Electrophoresis was performed on cellulose acetate after concentration
as previously described (Schuller, et al, 1969)

RESULTS

CSF protein values are given in Tables I and II. CSF
analysis of both patients showed a typical oligoclonal pattern (presence of 2 or 3 bands in gamma zone). In case 1,
important disturbance of the blood-CSF barrier seems associated because of the elevated CSF albumin.

In case 2, on the other hand, there is no transsudation.
In other words, the CSF pattern could be classified as a
"meningitic" pattern in the first case and as an "inflammatory" pattern in the second case (Schuller and Sagar, 1980)
Increase of alpha 1 globulin in CSF was found in 3/4 of all
assays.

DISCUSSION

The oligoclonal pattern of CSF protein electrophoresis
had never been reported untill recently in Alzheimer's
disease and senile dementia of the Alzheimer type. It had
not been found by Bock (1974) in her study on 16 demented
patients. In our experience, it has never been seen either
in the classical form of Alzheimer's disease or in Creutz-
feldt-Jakob disease. However, Williams, et al (1980) found
three abnormal bands in the CSF gamma-globulin region in five out of eight clinically diagnosed cases of Alzheimer's
disease. The oligoclonal CSF pattern is thought to be the
expression of IgG local synthesis. This has been demonstrated in patients with multiple sclerosis and subacute scle-
rosing panencephalitis by CSF electrophoresis and, more
precisely, by isoelectric focusing and isotachophoresis.
The alpha 1 increase in 3/4 CSF assays may be linked to so
called amyloid P component, an alpha 1 glycoprotein present
in normal serum and found in amyloid, mixed with various
types of amyloid proteins.

Whatever the nosological entity in which it is observed : classical Alzheimer disease and/or senile dementia
of the Alzheimer type or other disorders some of which could
represent a special clinicopathological entity, such as
emphasized particularly by Okazaki, et al (1979), the mechanism of amyloid deposit in the brain is discussed. It
might be produced by neurites or phagocytic cells themselves, which are present in senile plaques. It might, on
the contrary, especially in amyloid angiopathy, be secondary to a plasmatic transsudation (Ishii, et al, 1975,
Glenner, 1978, 1979). Our findings could support a third
hypothesis : a local abnormal immunoglobulin synthesis

208

could lead to the local production of an amyloidogenic protein. This could be either a short duration or a mild and
slow phenomenon. It could thus account for the absence of
the CSF oligoclonal pattern in classical form of Alzheimer'
s disease and the presence of such a pattern in some diseases with cerebral amyloid deposition.

AKNOWLEDGEMENTS

We thank Prs P.Castaigne, F.Lhermitte and J.L.Signoret
who provided us with clinical informations on their patients
and Dr E.Collum who kindly reviewed the English manuscript.

TABLE I - AMYLOID ANGIOPATHY : CSF PROTEINS OF PATIENT 1

	1	2	3
CSF total Protein(g/1)	0.95	1.40	1.33
Electro-phoresis	%	%	%
p A	3	2	2
A	44 (418 mg/1)	54 (756 mg/1)	56 (745 mg/1)
α 1	6 + 5	8	5
α 2	6	6	5
β 1	12	12	11
β 2	7	3	3
γ	6+11 (57+105mg/1)	5+10 (70+140mg/1)	8+6+4 (106+80+53 mg/1)

Conclusion : - association of IgG local synthesis (oligoclonal patterns : two or three bands in gamma zone, the value
of which is indicated) and transudation in the 3 CSF.
                - increase of α 1 in the two first CSF.

TABLE II - AMYLOID ANGIOPATHY : CSF PROTEINS OF PATIENT II

Electrophoresis	%	mg/l
p A	6	29
A	46	221
α 1	8	38
α 2	2	10
β 1	13	62
β 2	10	48
γ	6+9	29+43

Conclusion : - inflammatory CSF (no abnormal blood-brain barrier) with oligoclonal aspect (two bands, the value of which is indicated)

- light increase of α 1

REFERENCES

Bock, E., Kristensen, V., Rafaelsen, O.J.: Proteins in serum and cerebrospinal fluid in demented patients. Acta Neurol.Scandinav.50: 91-102, 1974.

Escourolle, R., and Poirier, J. : Manuel élémentaire de Neuropathologie (Masson, Paris 1976)

Glenner, G.G. : Current knowledge of amyloid deposits as applied to senile plaques and congophilic angopathy, in Alzheimer's disease : senile dementia and related disorders (Aging Vol.7) Ed.R.Klatzman, R.D. Terry and K.L.Bick, pp 493-501 (Raven Press, New-York 1978)

Glenner G.G. : Congophilic microangiopathy in the pathogenesis of Alzheimer's syndrome (presenil dementia). Medic.Hypoth.5: 1231-1236, 1979.

Gudmundsson, G., Hallgrimsson, J., Jonasson, T.A. and Bjarnason, O. : Hereditary cerebral hemorrhage with amyloidosis. Brain, 95: 387-404, 1972.

Ishii, T., Haga, S., Shimizu, F. : Identification of components of immunoglobulins in senile plaques by means of fluorescent antibody technique. Acta Neuropathol (Berl) 32: 157-162, 1975.

Jellinger, K. : Cerebrovascular amyloidosis with cerebral hemorrhage. J.Neurol.214: 195-206, 1977.

Katenkamp, D., Stiller, D., , : Comparisons of the texture of
     amyloid, collagen and Alzheimer cells. A polarisation
     micorscopic-histochemical study. Virchows Arch.Abt.
     A.Path.Anat. 359: 213-222, 1973.
Lee, S.S., Stemmermann, G.N. : Congophilic angiopathy and
     cerebral hemorrhage. Arch.Path.Lab.Med. 102: 317-321
     1978.
Linke, R.P. : Emerging classification of generalized and
     local amyloid deposits. In Recent Advances in Geron-
     tology. Ed.H.Orimo, K.Shimada, M.Iriki and D.Maeda,
     pp 464-469 (Excerpta Medica, Amsterdam, 1978)
Okazaki, H., Reagan, T.J., Campbell, R.J. : Clinicopatholo-
     gic studies of primary cerebral amyloid angiopathy.
     Mayo Clin.Proc. 54: 22-31, 1979.
Powers, J.M., Spicer, S.S. : Histochemical similarity of
     senile plaque amyloid to apudamyloid. Virchows Arch.
     Abt. A. Path.Anat. 376: 107-118, 1977.
Schuller, E., Rouques, C., Loridan, M. : Das Eiweisspektrum
     des Liquors im Verlauf der Multiplen Sklerose. Wien.
     Z.Nervenheilk (Supplt.II - 1969) 104.
Schuller, E., Sagar, H. : Local synthesis of CSF Immunoglo-
     bulins : a neuroimmunological classification. J.Neurol.
     Sci.1981, sous presse.
Williams, A., Papadopoulos, N., Chase, T.N. : Demonstration
     of CSF gamma-globulin banding in presenile dementia.
     Neurology, 30: 882-884, 1980.

POLYMORPHONUCLEAR FUNCTIONS

IN AGING ADULT HUMANS

J. Corberand, M.D. ; F. Nguyen, M.D. ; P. Laharrague, M.D.

A.M. Fontanilles, B. Gleyzes, E. Girard and C. Sénégas

Groupe d'Etude de la Phagocytose, Laboratoire d'Hématologie

C.H.U. Rangueil 31 054 Toulouse, and Unité 100 I.N.S.E.R.M

C.H.U. Purpan 31059 Toulouse FRANCE

ABSTRACT

Six tests of Polymorphonuclear leukocytes (PMNS) functions were performed in 217 healthy adults sub -classed by age into 7 groups including an equal number of males and females. The functional properties of PMNS in the aged, when compared to those of the younger adults were characterized by a decrease of the chemotactic response in the group "over 80", an increased adherence over 70 years, a progressive decrease of the NBT reduction capability, and a diminished Candida killing activity appearing in the over 60 years group. Spontaneous migration and phagocytosis were unaffected. Such an impairement may contribute to the well known susceptibility to bacterial infection which affects the aged.

INTRODUCTION

Neutrophil polymorphonuclear leukocytes (PMNS) constitute a first line barrier against infective organisms (GALLIN and QUIE, I978). Much is presently known concerning the relationships between various functional defects of these blood cells and infection (STOSSEL and COHEN, I977). The influence of age on PMN function has already been reported in newborn babies whose chemotactic and bactericidal activities are diminished when compared to adult's (MILLER,I971 ; COEN, et al., I969). The present study was undertaken to verify if normal aging does interfere with the functional capability of PMNS in adults.

MATERIALS AND METHODS

Venous blood was obtained from 285 autonomous and informed volunteers aged from 20 to 97 years and considered as being healthy. Subjects with diseases capable of altering PMN functions, such as diabetes mellitus, rheumatoid arthritis or tuberculosis, were rejected from the study, as well as those currently or recently infected subjects or those individuals under treatment whatever the reason, oral contraceptives excepted. Along with the PMNs' study, several blood parameters (blood cell enumeration and differential, ESR, sugar, creatinine and nitrogen) were measured. Those subjects who demonstrated at least one abnormality were eliminated from the study. The medical history of over 70 years subjects was reviewed after a six months interval. Their results were validated in the absence of any pathological event during the elapsed period. Using these criteria, 68 series of PMNS functions results had to be rejected. The 217 remaining subjects were sub -classed by age into 7 groups (Table 1). Each group corresponded to a 10 years period, with the exception of the last one (over 80) where 8 individuals (5 males, 3 females) were over 90 years old. The study was carried out during a 27 month period. Subjects in the different groups were not studied simultaneously, as the recruitment of true healthy individuals over 60 years of age was most difficult.

TABLE 1 - AGE AND SEX DISTRIBUTIONS OF SUBJECTS STUDIED FOR FUNCTIONAL PMN ACTIVITY

Age groups in years	20-29	30-39	40-49	50-59	60-69	70-79	>80
Mean age	24.4	34.1	45.2	54.9	65.2	73.7	86.8
($\pm$ 1 S.D*)	$\pm$2.7	$\pm$2.2	$\pm$2.5	$\pm$3.0	$\pm$2.7	$\pm$2.6	$\pm$4.4
Number of subjects	31	34	32	30	30	31	29
– Males	15	18	15	15	15	15	13
– Females	16	16	17	15	15	16	16

*Standard Deviation.

Six functional PMN tests were simultaneously performed in each subject. They were :

.Capillary tube random migration according the whole blood method of KETCHELL (KETCHELL and FAVOUR, 1955).Heparinated whole blood was centrifuged in ten capillary tubes and vertically incubated for 4 hours. The distance between the front of leukocytes and the erythrocytes level was measured microscopically on each tube. The result was expressed as the arithmetic mean of the distances measured in the ten tubes.

.Chemotaxis under agarose using the method of NELSON (NELSON, et al 1975). Two distances were microscopically measured, representing the spontaneous migration (B) and the chemotactic response to the zymosan activated autologous serum(A). The results were expressed as a chemotactic index (A/B ratio).

.Adherence to nylon fibers according to the method of ZITTOUN (ZITTOUN and BERCHE, 1973). The absolute numbers of PMN$_s$ were determined before and after filtration of 5 ml blood through sixty milligrams of scrubbed nylon packed into 20 ml glass syringes. The results were expressed as the percentage of PMN$_s$ retained during filtration.

.Particle ingestion activity was expressed by the Phagocytic Index according to BRANDT's technique (BRANDT, 1967). A suspension of heat killed yeast cells was added to a leukocyte suspension to obtain a ratio of 8 yeast cells : 1 PMN. After incubation the number of PMN$_s$ which had ingested yeast particles was established microscopically on stained smears. The score obtained for 100 consecutive PMN$_s$ divided by 100 provided the Phagocytic Index.

.Nitroblue Tetrazolium (NBT) dye reduction was studied according to the quantitative technique reported by BAEHNER (BAEHNER and NATHAN,1968). Two assays were carried out in parallel, one for the spontaneous reduction of NBT by PMN$_s$, the other for the NBT reduction by PMN$_s$ phagocytosing latex particles. The reduced NBT was extracted in the presence of pyridine and spectrophotometrically measured at 515 nm. The results were expressed as resting O D (optical density) for resting PMN$_s$ and latex OD for stimulated PMN$_s$. The Δ O Ddifference between the two previous values, represented the potential of metabolic stimulation of the phagocytes.

.Candida Killing activity was studied using the method of LEHRER (LEHRER and CLINE, 1969). A leukocyte suspension was incubated with pooled AB serum opsonized candida albicans grown in the yeast phase. Thereafter, the leukocytes were disrupted by addition of 2.5% sodium deoxycholate (MERCK, Darmstadt, West Germany). The percentage of killed candida was established using the dye exclusion method with methylene blue. A control tube containing no leukocytes was carried out in parallel. The results of the candida killing activity, expressed as the percentage of stained yeasts, was obtained by substracting the percentage obtained in the control tube from that of the reaction tube.

.Statistical data : comparison of the means was interpreted according the student's t test. The differences were considered to be significant when the probability (p) was < 0.05.

RESULTS

The results of the six tests exploring the functions of PMN$_s$ are
shown for each group in table 2.

TABLE 2 - RESULTS OF THE SIX PMNs' FUNCTIONAL TESTS ACCORDING TO THE
AGE GROUPS (mean ± 1 standard deviation)

Age groups in years	20-29	30-39	40-49	50-59	60-69	70-79	>80
Random migration	1.99 ±0.25	1.87 ±0.24	1.89 ±0.22	1.88 ±0.27	1.94 ±0.37	1.95 ±0.46	1.94 ±0.47
Chemotaxis	1.64 ±0.23	1.67 ±0.16	1.61 ±0.14	1.70 ±0.25	1.71 ±0.22	1.68 ±0.23	1.58 ±0.15
Adherence	69.8 ±9.6	72.3 ±12.6	68.5 ±12.5	67.2 ±14.1	69.3 ±15.5	73.1 ±16.2	79.7 ±15.7
Phagocytosis	4.34 ±0.56	4.70 ±0.49	4.71 ±0.50	4.63 ±0.64	4.79 ±0.66	4.78 ±0.59	4.54 ±0.61
NBT reduction (ΔOD)	0.384 ±0.064	0.341 ±0.049	0.348 ±0.055	0.341 ±0.070	0.304 ±0.089	0.274 ±0.048	0.328 ±0.090
Candida killing	31.4 ±2.7	31.7 ±2.9	30.5 ±2.9	31.8 ±2.5	29.1 ±3.6	29.6 ±4.3	27.8 ±3.5

The only statistically significant difference in PMN chemotaxis
appears in the "over 80" group. The mean value is lower than that of the
group constituted by the rest of the studied population (20-79 years),
whose value was 1.66 ±0.20 (p <0.01). This difference depends only on
the reponse of PMNs to the chemotactic stimulus since no variation was
observed in the spontaneous migration under agarose with age.

Results of PMN adherence did not very among the first six groups.
In the group "over 80" the mean value was the highest, the value being
statistically increased when compared to each group between 20 and 69
years.

The result in the "70-79" group was intermediate between the 6 first group and the last one.

The results of the PMN phagocytosis presented no difference from a group to an other over 30 years. The lowest value was obtained in the youngest group. However, it should be noted that their result was not stastistically different from those of the "50-59" and "over 80" groups.

The Δ OD results of the NBT reduction test were observed to decrease with age with the exception of the "over 80 years" (fig.1). The evolution of the stimulated OD values were similar. Conversely, the values of resting OD were grossly increasing with age. In the "over 80" group the Δ OD value rose to a level comparable to that of the "50-59" and "60-69" groups, but remained lower than that of the youngest group ($p < 0,01$).

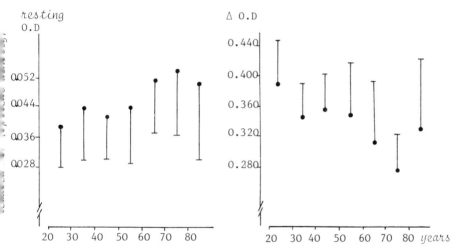

Figure 1 : Evolution of the NBT reduction capability of resting and stimulated PMN$_s$ according to age. The black circles and the vertical bars represent respectively the mean and one standard deviation for each age group.

As for the candida killing capacity, no linear correlation could be found with the age. However, there exists a statistically significant difference ($p < 0.001$) between the group of 125 subjects aged 20 to 59 (31.4 ± 2.7) and the group of 90 subjects aged over 60 years (28.8 ± 3.9) the lowest value being observed in the older group (fig.2).

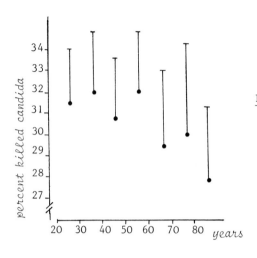

Figure 2 : Evolution of candida killing activity according to age.
The mean values for the two groups "20-59" and "60-89" years are plotted as horizontal bars.

No variation according the age group was observed in the capillary tube random migration test. Nevertheless, il should be noted that the standard deviations of the means were wider in the over 60 years groups than in the youngers.

CONCLUSIONS

The long lifespan of humans prevented us from using a longitudinal study as it can be done in animal models. Therefore we chose to study a large population of adults selected according to clinical and biological criteria as being healthy and unmedicated, that latter disposition being considered as strictly important. Thus 68 subjects, representing 24 % of the initial recruited population, had to be rejected, principally in the older groups, mostly because continuing medication.

The functional tests were selected to explore the principal functions of PMN$_S$. Thus, the migratory properties, spontaneous and stimulated, the phagocytic capacity, the metabolic stimulation which produces potent microbicidal agents, and one aspect of the microbicidal activity expressed in the present work as the candida killing activity, all properties which constitute the basic steps of PMN function, were tested.

To our knowledge, no comparable study, have been previously performed on such a diverse populations. Only a few references exist in the literature. PHAIR et al (1978) found a defect of chemotaxis in 7 % of volunteers aged over 65 years. This result is very similar to ours since only 4 subjects of our oldest group had individual values below one

standard deviation of the mean obtained from the "20-79 years" group.
An increase of adherence has been previously described by SILVERMAN and
SILVERMAN (1977), but conversely to our results the increase was observed in subjects over 60 years and a difference appeared between males
and females. Whereas we witnessed no variation in phagocytosis using
saccharomyces cerevisiae, the function was reported to be impaired in
the aged by MORONI et al (1976) and IVANOVA (1978). Bacteria was used
in those two studies. Conflicting results have been published concerning the bacterial killing by PMNs in aged subsjects, either normal
(MORONI, et al, 1975 ; PALMBLAD and HAAK, 1978) or diminished (PHAIR et
al, 1978). However it should be noted that in the latter report, the
impairment was found in only 8 subjects (11 % of the studied population) and was only transient. In our study, candida killing activity
was concerned and its decrease observed in the "over 60 years" group,
affected 37 % of that population. As for the NBT reduction, the impairment described by MORONI et al (1975) affected only the subsjects older
than 60 years and presenting with auto-antibodies.

The impairment of the NBT reduction, characterized by a progressive
decreased of stimulated OD paralleled by a progressive and proportional
increase of resting OD, that we observed in our work, is similar to
what has been previously observed in rheumatoïd arthritis (CORBERAND et
al, 1977a) and malignant lymphomas (CORBERAND et al, 1977b).

Humoral factors are suspected to interfere with circulating PMNs
(JOHNSTON and LEHMEYER, 1976) in these conditions. Nevertheless, the increase of stimulated NBT reduction we observed in our oldest group remains unexplained and suggests the involvement of additional "extra-
aging factor". This factor should not be a latent infection since no
change was observed in the absolute PMNs number, the ESR and the neutrophil alkaline phosphatase score.

Our findings as well as those of the above cited authors confirm
that PMN functions are impaired in the elderly. The age of appearance
varies, according to the function, between the sixties and the eighties.
As for other human physiological functions, these anomalies are subject
to individual variations.

The mechanisms by which this impairment occurs are hypothetical.
Two possibilities may be proposed :

(a) an intrinsic defect of PMN$_S$ pre-existing to their arrival in the
blood stream. (b) an acquired abnormality due to the action of components whose appearance in the plasma depends itself on the aging process. These factors might be by-products of the defective metabolisms
(MICHELSON, 1976 ; HARMAN et al, 1977 ; RIVNAY et al, 1979) or the products of immunological disturbances (LANGE, 1977) such as auto-antibodies or circulating immune complexes. In this way the defective PMN may
be only a victim of the aging process.

REFERENCES

Baehner, R.L., Nathan D.G.: Quantitative nitroblue tetrazolium test in
    chronic granulomatous disease. New. Engl. J. Med. 278 : 971, 1968.
Brandt L. : Studies on the phagocytic activity of neutrophilic leuko-
    cytes. Scand. J. Haematol. suppl. 2 : 1, 1967.
Coen R., Grush O., Kauder E. : Studies of bactericidal activity and me-
    tabolism of the leukocytes in full term neonates. J. Pediatr. 75 :
    400, 1969.
Corberand J., Amigues H., De Larrard B. : Neutrophil function in rheu-
    matoid arthritis. Scand. J. Rheumatol. 6 : 49, 1977.
Corberand J., Benchekroun S., Biermé R. : Neutrophil function in mali-
    gnant lymphoma. Communication : Fourth Meeting Intern. Soc. Hae-
    matology. Istambul September 1977.
Gallin J.I. and Quie P.G. : Leukocyte chemotaxis : Methods, physiology
    and clinical implications. Raven Press. New York 1978.
Harman D., Heidrick M.L., Eddy D.E. : Free radical theory of aging :
    effect of free-radical-reaction inhibitors on the immune response.
    J. Am. Geriatrics Soc. 25 : 400, 1977.
Inova N.I. : Age characteristics of the phagocytic reaction of neutro-
    phils. Vrach. Delo. 5 : 49, 1978.
Johnston R.B., Lehmeyer J.E. : Elaboration of toxic oxygen by-products
    by neutrophils in a model of immune complex disease. J. Clin. In-
    vest. 57 : 836, 1976.
Ketchel M.M., Favour C.B. : The acceleration and inhibition of migra-
    tion on human leukocytes in vitro by plasma protein fractions.
    J. Exp. Med. 101 : 647, 1955.
Lange C.F. : Immunology of aging. in "Progress in clinical pathology,
    vol VII, ed. by Stefanini M. , New York, Grune et Stratton, 1977,
    p. 119.
Lehrer R.I., Cline M.J. : Interaction of candida albicans with human
    leukocytes and serum. J. Bact. 98 : 996, 1969.
Michelson A.M. : Rôle biologique du radical anion superoxyde et des
    superoxyde-dismutases dans le métabolisme cellulaire. C.R. Soc.
    Biol. Paris, 170 : 1137, 1976.
Miller M.E. : Chemotactic function in the human neonate : humoral and
    cellular aspects. Pediatr. Res. 5 : 487, 1971.
Moroni M., Capsoni F., Caredda F., Lazzarin A., Basana C. : Demonstra-
    tion of a granulocyte defect in aged persons correlated with the
    presence of auto-antibodies. Boll. Inst. Sieroter. Milano. 55 :
    317, 1976.

Nelson R.D., Quie P.G., Simmons R.L. : Chemotaxis under agarose : a new and simple method for measuring chemotaxis and spontaneous migration of human polyporphonuclear leukocytes and monocytes. J. Immunol. 115 : 1650, 1975.

Palmblad J., Haak A. : Ageing does not change blood granulocyte bactericidal capacity and levels of complement factors 3 and 4. Gerontology, 24 : 381, 1978.

Phair J.P., Kauffman C.A., Bjornson A., Gallagher J., Adams L., Hess E.V Host defenses in the aged : evaluation of components of the inflammatory and immune responses. J. Infect. Dis. 138 : 67, 1978.

Rivnay B., Globerson A., Shinitzky M. : Viscosity of lymphocyte plasma membrane in aging mice and its possible relation to serum cholesterol. Mech. Ageing. Develop. 10 : 71, 1979.

Silverman E.M., Silverman A.G. : Granulocyte adherence in the elderly. Am. J. Clin. Pathol. 67 : 49, 1977.

Stossel T.P., Cohen H.J. : Neutrophil functions : normal and abnormal. in "The year in hematology. Ed. by A.S. Gordon, R. Sibber, J. Lobue New York, Plenum medical book company, 1977, p. 191.

Zittoun R., Berche P.A. : L'adhésivité au verre et le pouvoir phagocytaire des polynucléaires neutrophiles dans les syndromes myéloprolifératifs et les anémies réfractaires. Path. Biol. Paris 21 : 271, 1973.

INFLUENCE OF SUPPLEMENTAL ORAL ZINC ON THE IMMUNE RESPONSE OF OLD PEOPLE

Jean Duchateau, Guy Delespesse and Max Kunstler

Department of Immuno-allergology, Hôpital Universitaire Saint-Pierre

and Institut Pacheco, Bruxelles, Belgium.

ABSTRACT

Oral zinc was given to 12 healthy subjects over 70 years old (220 mg zinc sulfate, twice a day for one month) compared to 12 controls, matched for age and sex, and simultaneously tested. The following changes were attributed to zinc treatment : an increase of T cells but not B cells numbers, an improvement of positivity and intensity of delayed skin reactions to 3 common antigens. In vitro lymphocyte proliferative responses to 3 mitogens remained depressed in both groups. All subjects were then challenged with tetanos toxoid vaccine. Their in vivo and in vitro specific IgG antibody production was measured before and 3 weeks after the vaccination. Zinc pretreatment improved clearly the serum rise of specific antibodies to tetanos toxin, as well as their in vitro production in Pokeweed Mitogen stimulated cultures. The same experimental design was used for two groups of 10 healthy young people 23-45 years old receiving 200 mg zinc acetate or placebo (twice a day, one month) in double blind, then vaccinated and tested identically. Starting levels and rise of antibodies were considerably higher than in elderly but unaffected by zinc. It is suggested that oral zinc increases differentiation of T cell and the limited helper interactions rather than proliferative in aged people, without modifying more optimal responses of younger.

INTRODUCTION

Animal experiments have shown that selective zinc deficiency leads to profound alterations of several parameters of T cells function such as atrophy of the thymus and severe impairment of T cells helper and cytotoxic activities. All these features are reversible after zinc repletion (reviewed in Good et al., 1979). Similar observations linking immune abnormalities with zinc deficiency and restoration after zinc supplementation are now documented in human clinical conditions. This is the case for acrodermatitis enteropathica (Endre et al., 1975; Julius et al., 1973), total parenteral nutrition (Pekarek et al., 1979), protein calorie malnutrition (Golden et al., 1977; Golden et al., 1978) and Down's syndrome (Björksten et al., 1980).

Aging is associated with a progressive thymic involution and alteration of immune competence affecting mainly but not exclusively T lymphocyte function (reviewed in Makinodan and Kay, 1980).

Serum and hair zinc levels decrease 20 to 30 % from the age of 12
to over 70 years (reviewed in Hsu, 1979) although red cells concentrations is stable (Lindeman et al, 1971). Wether true zinc deficiency
occurs with aging is not established but undirectly suggested by dietary
investigations in aged people (Greger and Sciscoe, ·1977). We have shown
that oral zinc could enhance lymphocyte mitogen responses of young
healthy people, an effect depending on the initial level of individual
response (Duchateau et al., 1981). Owing to the safety of oral zinc
sulfate administration in geriatric patients (Czerwinsky et al., 1973)
we decided to investigate its influence on the compromised immune status
of old people.

We report here the effect of oral zinc supplementation on the following immune parameters : circulating T cells, in vitro lymphocyte response to mitogens delayed skin reactions. We also compare the influence
of supplemental zinc administration on the in vitro and in vivo IgG antibody production after tetanos toxoid vaccination in young and old subjects.

MATERIAL AND METHODS

Participants :

1) two groups of 12 age and sex paired institutionalized people, aged
   over 70 years were selected for their healthy conditions. Affectation
   to treatment was randomized and the treated group received 220 mg
   zinc sulfate twice a day for one month. The other received no placebo. Care was taken to manage the two groups in identical way and
   equal numbers of each were tested simultaneously and in blind.

2) two groups of 10 healthy young people, matched for age (23-45) and
   sex were given 200 mg zinc acetate or placebo twice a day for one
   month in a double blind procedure.

Lymphocyte studies : briefly, lymphocytes were separated from hepari-
nized venous blood by density gradient centrifugation on Ficoll-Urogra-
phine, washed in hanks balanced salt solution (Ca and Mg free : Gibco-
Biocult). T cells were determined by their ability to form E rosettes
according to the method of Jondal, Holme and Wigzell (1972).

B cells were identified as immunoglobulin bearing cells by a direct
fluorescent assay (Preud'homme and Flandrin, 1974). Lymphocyte cultures
were performed as previously described (Delespesse et al., 1976) in RPMI
1640 (Flow Lab) supplemented with 10 % AB human serum, 5 mM glutamine,
40 μg/ml gentamycine; they were stimulated with purified phytohemagglutinin (PHA-P, Welcome Lab) 1 μg/ml, Concavanalin A (Con A, Miles Lab)
or pokeweed mitogen 1/100 (PWM, Gibco-Biocult). Proliferation was measured by the uptake of tritiated thymidine (5 μC - 10 C/mM) added 18
hours before harvesting on day three. IgG antibody specific for tetanos
toxin was measured in the supernatant of 6 days lymphocyte cultures stimulated with PWM 1/100 in the presence of fetal calf serum (10 %). IgG
anti-tetanos were determined by the same radioimmunoassay as for serum.
Skin tests : intradermal injections of 0.1 ml of the following solutions
were made in the forearm : Candidin (Beecham : dilution 0.5 %), Streptokinase-Streptodornase (Varidase : Lederle 10 U/0.1 ml) and purified
protein derivative (PPD : Statens Serum Inst. Denmark 2 U/0.1 ml). The
same batches were used at one month interval. Induration diameters were
measured 48 hours after injection by the same observer ignorant of the
individual treatment.

Antibody response to tetanos toxoid vaccination

After one month of zinc treatment all groups received an intramuscular
injection of tetanos toxoid (0.5 ml, Tevax : RIT, Genval). Serum was
taken before the vaccination and 3 weeks later. Specific IgG antibodies
were measured by a solid phase radioassay (Delespesse et al., 1979).
Tetanos toxin (TT) coated polystyrene microtubes were incubated overnight at room temperature with 200 μl of test serum diluted 1/40. The
tubes were washed and then further incubated during six hours with
200 μl ^{125}I protein A from staphylococcal Aureus (Pharmacia, Sweden).
After several washes, the remaining radioactivity was counted, and taken
as a measure of IgG anti TT antibodies. Titers were determined by reference to a standard curve made of serial two fold dilutions of an hyperimmune serum considered to titer 1024 arbitrary units. Blanks were
obtained using a serum from a non immune young healthy subject.

RESULTS

Mean age of elderly treated group was 81 $\pm$ 4 and 79 $\pm$ 5 for untreated (mean $\pm$ SD). Both included 6 women and 6 men.

Lymphocytes and mitogen responses :

Table 1 summarizes data on identification of circulating lymphocytes and
their mitogen stimulations for each group, before (I) and after (II) zinc
treatment. Although mean lymphocyte counts remained stable (1980 $\pm$ 560)
in all the tests the proportion of E rosette forming cells raised significantly in the treated subjects (p < 0.05 paired T test) whereas Ig
bearing cells remained unchanged. As a consequence, the proportions of
non T, non B lymphocytes were decreased. Mitogen stimulations with PHA,
Con A and PWM were reduced to almost half of that from two young people
simultaneously and repeatly tested. Relative values were not different
after one month, in both groups wether treated or not.

Table 1 - LYMPHOCYTE IDENTIFICATION AND MITOGEN RESPONSE

Groups	Lymphocyte subsets			Mitogen stimulation		
	T	B	NI	PHA	Con A	PWM
Treated						
I	72 %	9 %	19 %	38 $\pm$ 6 %	51 $\pm$ 7 %	53 $\pm$ 8 %
II	79	11	10	40 $\pm$ 7	47 $\pm$ 7	76 $\pm$ 18
	p < 0.05 (paired T)		p < 0.05 (X^2)			
Untreated						
I	71	11	18	50 $\pm$ 7	56 $\pm$ 14	47 $\pm$ 15
II	72	11	17	50 $\pm$ 12	62 $\pm$ 17	68 $\pm$ 8
Young controls						
I	100 %			267	170	118
II	100 %			304	193	99

This represents mean % of characterized lymphocyte subsets among
zinc treated or untreated aged people at first (I) and second (II)
bleeding : E rosettes (T), surface Ig bearing cells (B) and non
identified (NI) lymphocytes. Peroxydase positive cells were excluded.
Mitogen stimulation is expressed as mean percentage $\pm$ SEM from mean
values of two young men (34 and 35 year old) who were simultaneously
and repeatedly (3 x) tested as internal controls at each assay. Their
results are expressed as mean net CPM x 10^{-3} at the bottom of the table.

Skin tests : a reaction was considered as positive if mean diameter of
induration was ⩾ 5 mm; it was classified as negative if the diameter was
⩽ 2 mm and doubtfull if the diameter was comprised between 2 and 5 mm.
Although basic distributions were similar in both groups the net result
after one month zinc treatment was a straight reduction of the frequency
of negative responses and a raise of positive one in the treated group
(Table 2). No significant change occured in the other group.
By summing the indurations diameters to the three antigens we obtained
a score that was representative of individual intensity of delayed type
response. This dramatically enhanced to almost the double of initial
value (p < 0.01 paired T test) in the treated group whereas only slightly
increased at a non significantly level in the control group (Table 2,
right part).

Table 2 - DELAYED TYPE SKIN REACTIONS

Groups (n = 12	Induration < 2 mm	⩾ 5 mm		Mean individual score (sum of 3 tests)	
Treated					
I	14	16		18 ± 3.9	
II	6	26	p < 0.01 (x^2)	35.3 ± 5.6	p < 0.01 (paired T test)
Untreated					
I	11	17		16 ± 3.6	
II	13	19	NS	20 ± 5.5	NS

The left part of the table shows the cumulated frequency of skin
responses to candidin, streptokinase-streptodornase and PPD among
the treated and untreated aged people in function of their induration
diameters (36 tests) before (I) and after (II) one month.
On the right part are the mean scores ± SEM of individual sum of the
3 recorded induration diameters (n = 12).

In vitro anti-tetanos toxin IgG antibody production :

At the completion of zinc treatment the production of IgG anti TT (IgG-a-TT) antibodies was measured before and 3 weeks after vaccination. As shown in figure 1 A the mean IgG a-TT production was higher after than before vaccination. The increase of the in vitro antibody synthesis was more pronounced in the zinc treated subjects. The influence of zinc on these parameters was even more apparent when individuals with the same starting levels (< 15 U) of antibody synthesis were compared (figure 1 B, $p < 0.05$ paired Wilcoxon test).

In vivo anti TT IgG antibody response (figure 2) :

In young people zinc treatment had no influence on IgG a-TT response. Note that 3 participants treated with placebo were not included in this figure because they appeared to be hyperimmunized and did not respond to the present vaccination. The prevaccination levels of old subjects were five fold lower than those of the younger group. Untreated old

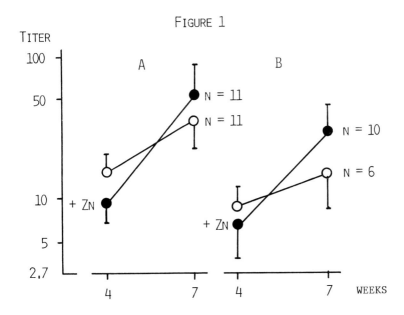

FIGURE 1

In vitro production of specific IgG a-TT antibody in old subjects treated or not with zinc, before and after vaccination.

people displayed only a two fold increase of their antibody titer as opposed to a ten fold increase in the treated subjects (p < 0.05 paired T test).

DISCUSSION

The present study shows clearly the beneficial influence of zinc supplementation on several parameters of cellular immunity in aged people :

1) increase of detectable circulating T cells at expense of non identified lymphocytes, whereas B cells number was stable.
2) enhancement of delayed type hypersensitivity to common antigens.
3) amelioration of specific IgG antibodies production in vivo and in

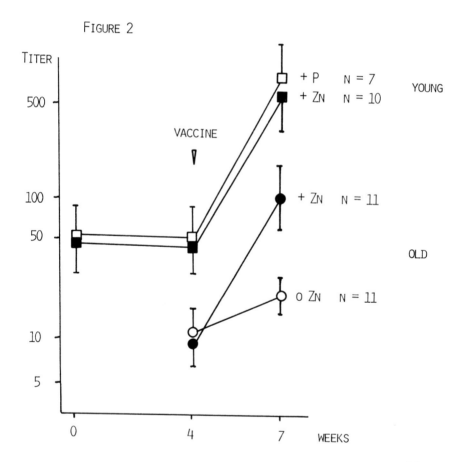

FIGURE 2

Serum specific IgG a-TT antibodies level in young and old subjects treated or not with zinc, before and after TT vaccine.

vitro after tetanos toxoid vaccination. The depressed mitogen proliferative response to PHA, Con A and PWM were unaffected.

This seems to indicate that zinc treatment favorized more importantly the differentiation and/or the cellular interactions than the
cellular proliferation itself, leading to more effective help from T
cells. The mode of action is unknown.

Correction of marginal zinc deficiency is not excluded but seems
unlikely. Although serum or hair levels of zinc were not available in
old participants of this study, there was no clinical signs of deficiency
(anosmia, anorexia, etc...) and their diet was controlled by dieteti-
cians. Reported data in the literature based on determination of serum
and hair concentration in zinc suggest a marginal zinc deficiency in the
elderly. However, this view is challenged by the finding of a significant overlapping between values obtained in adults and old subjects.

More critical seems to be the zinc availability at the site of
inflammation as evidenced by our observation (in preparation) of a beneficial effect of zinc ointment on the delayed skin response.

Increased delayed skin reactions and antibody response could be
secondary to the influence of supplemental zinc on circulating T cells.
This might be due to a thymic effect as suggested by the report of
change in levels of thymic hormones in some immunodeficient patients
treated with oral zinc (Cunningham-Rundle et al., 1979). Furthermore,
addition of zinc to normal mice diet leads to a delayed decay of Facteur Thymique Serique levels with aging (Iwata et al., 1979). Attempts
to correct antibody forming capacity of old spleen cells succeeded par-
tialy in mice through injection of thymopoietin prepared by C. Goldstein
(Weksler et al., 1978) when others (Martinez et al., 1978) with similar
preparation ubiquitin or FTS failed to correct their T cell mitogenic
response and resistance to tumor cells. The last point excepted this
is the pattern of positive and negative effects we observed in our old
subjects.

Zinc could also modify lymphocyte traffic which is controlled by
metal binding proteins (De Sousa, 1978). Activated lymphocytes have
receptors for transferrin and zinc transferrin (Galbraith, 1980 and our
own, to be published). We have shown that zinc could modify transferrin
binding to lymphocytes (Duchateau et al., 1980). Wether some different
zinc saturation of transferrin could influence lymphocyte localization
is only suggested by the above mentioned experiments with topical zinc

application and remains to be demonstrated.

A direct effect of zinc on cellular membrane is not excluded.
Zinc treatment of humans with sickle cells anemia impete the sickling
process (Brewer et al., 1978). In animals, in vivo zinc administrations
is able to inhibit macrophage migration and function (reviewed in
Chvapil, 1976 and Chvapil et al., 1979). An increased activity of mononuclear phagocytes has been described in experimental animals during
aging and has been related to their reduced antibody response to small
dose of antigens (Heidrick, 1972).

The improvement of TT antibody response in the elderly under the
influence of zinc might be secondary to an effect on the T helper cell
function, which is altered during aging. This might explain the absence
of effect on the antibody production by the younger group where the
helper function is not limiting the IgG antibody synthesis.

REFERENCES

Björksten, B., Bäck, O., Gustavson, K.H., Hallmans, G., Hägglöf, B.
    and Tärnvik, A. : Zinc and immune function in Down's syndrome.
    Acta Pediat. Scand. 69 : 183-187, 1980.
Brewer, G.J., Brewer, L.F. and Prasad, A.S. : Suppression of irreversi-
    bly sickled erythrocytes by zinc therapy in sickle cell anemia.
    J. Lab. Clin. Med. 90 : 549-554, 1977.
Chvapil, M. : Effects of zinc on cells and biomembranes. Med. Clin.
    North Am. 60 : 799-812, 1976.
Chvapil, M., Stankova, L., Bartos, Z., Cox, T. and Nichols, W. :
    Mobility of peritoneal inflammatory cells after in vivo supplemen-
    tation with zinc. J. Reticuloendoth. Soc. 25 : 345-350, 1979.
Cunningham-Rundles, C., Cunningham-Rundles, S., Garafolo, J., Iwata, T.,
    Incefy, G., Twomey, J. and Good, R.A. : Increased T lymphocytes
    function and thymopoietin following zinc repletion in man.
    Fed. Proc. 38 : 1222, 1979.
Czerwinsky, A.W., Clark, M.L., Serafetinides, E.A., Perrier, C.B.A.
    and Huber, W.H. : Safety and efficacy of zinc sulfate in geriatric
    patients. Clin. Pharmacol. and Therap. 15 : 436-441, 1973.
Delespesse, G., Duchateau, J., Gausset, Ph. and Govaerts, A. : In vitro
    response of subpopulations of human tonsil lymphocytes. I. Cellular
    collaboration in the proliferative response to PHA and Con A.
    J. Immunol. 116 : 437-445, 1976.
de Sousa, M. : Lymphoid cell positionning : a new proposal for the
    mechanism of control of lymphoid cell migration. Symp. Soc. Exp.
    Biol. 32 : 393-410, 1978.
Duchateau, J., Delespesse, G., Collet, H. and De Koster, J. : Transferrin
    binding human lymphocytes detected by a rosette technique.
    (Abstract) Abstracts 4th international Congress of Immunology of
    the IUIS, Ed. J.L. Preud'homme and V.A.L. Hawken, pp. 20.8 (Paris,
    1980).
Duchateau, J., Delespesse, G. and Vereecke, P. : Influence of oral zinc
    supplementation on the lymphocyte response to mitogens of normal
    subjects. Am. J. Clin. Nutr., early issues in 1981.

Endre, L., Datona, Z. and Gyurkowits, L. : Zinc deficiency and cellular
    immune deficiency in acrodermatitis enteropathica. Lancet 7917 :
    1196, 1975.
Galbraith, G.M.P., Goust, J.M., Mercurio, S.M. and Galbraith, R.M. :
    Transferrin binding by mitogen activated human peripheral blood
    lymphocytes. Clin. Immunol. Immunopath. 16 : 387-395, 1980.
Golden, M.N.H., Jackson, A.A. and Golden, B.E. : Effect of zinc on
    thymus of malnourished children. Lancet 8047 : 1057-1059, 1977.
Golden, M.N.H., Golden, B.E., Harland, P.S.E.G. and Harland, A.A. :
    Zinc and immunocompetence in protein energy malnutrition. Lancet
    8076 : 1226-1228, 1978.
Good, R.A., Fernandez, G. and West, A. : Nutrition, immunologic aging
    and disease. Aging and immunity, Ed. Singhal, Sinclair and Stiller,
    pp. 141-163 (Elsevier North Holland, Amsterdam, 1979).
Greger, J.L. and Scicoe, B.S. : Zinc nutriture of elderly participants
    in an urban feeding program. Research 70 : 37-41, 1971.
Heidrick, M.L. : Age related changes in hydrolase activity of perito-
    neal macrophages. Gerontologist 12 : 28-35, 1972.
Hsu, J.M. : Current knowledge on zinc, copper and chromium in aging.
    Wld. Rev. Nutr. Diet. 33 : 42-69, 1979.
Iwata, T., Incefy, G.S., Tanaka, T., Fernandez, G., Menendez-Botet,
    C.J., Pih, K. and Good, R.A. : Circulating thymic hormone levels
    in zinc deficiency. Cell. Immunol. 47 : 100-105, 1979.
Jondal, M., Holm, G. and Wigzell, H.J. : Surface markers on human T
    and B lymphocytes. I. A large population of lymphocytes forming
    non immune rosettes with sheep red blood cells. J. Exp. Med. 136 :
    207-212, 1972.
Julius, R., Shulking, M., Psrinkle, T. and Rennert, O. : Acrodermatitis
    enteropathica with immune deficiency. J. Pediat. 83 : 1007-1011,
    1973.
Lindeman, R.D., Clark, M.L. and Calmore, J.P. : Influence of age and
    sex on plasma and red cell zinc concentration. J. Gerontol. 26 :
    358-363, 1971.
Makinodan, T. and Kay, M.B. : Age influence on the immune system.
    Adv. in Immunol. 29 : 287-330, 1980.
Martinez, D., Field, A.K., Schwam, H., Tytell, A.A. and Hilleman, M.R.
    Soc. Exp. Biol. Med. 159 : 195, cited in Makinodan 1980.
Pekarek, R.S., Sandstead, H.H., Facob, R.A. and Barcome, D.F. :
    Abnormal cellular immune responses during acquired zinc defi-
    ciency. Am. J. Clin. Nutr. 32 : 1466-1471, 1979.
Preud'homme, J.L. and Flandrin, G.J. : Identification by peroxydase
    staining of monocytes in surface immunofluorescence tests.
    J. Immunol. 113 : 1650-1658, 1974.
Weksler, M.E., Innes, J.B. and Goldstein, G. : Immunological studies of
    aging. IV. The contribution of thymic involution to the immune
    deficiencies of aging mice and reversal with thymopoietin 32-36.
    J. Exp. Med. 148 : 996-1006, 1978.